# NATUROPATHIC CANCER CARE

A Safe and Effective approach to healing

from Cancer

**John Byrne N.D., B.H.Sc.**

# DEDICATION

This book is dedicated to Beulah, who has been more than dedicated to me for 16 years.

May I be someday what she sees in me.

## BYRNE FAMILY PHOTO

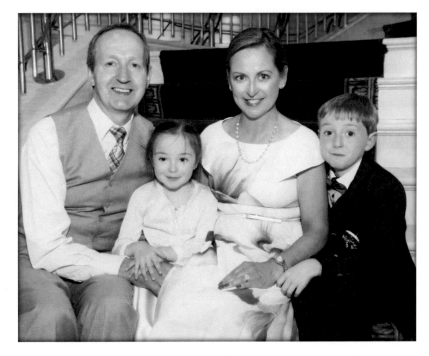

From left to right: John, Olivia, Beulah and Shane.

## About the Author

John Byrne N.D., B.H.Sc. is an accomplished Naturopath and author with over 20 year's post-graduate experience, study and personal research in the area of chronic disease including cancer. He has earned his Bachelor's degree in Health Science from the University of New England in NSW, along with an advanced diploma in Naturopathy, diplomas in Nutrition, Herbal Medicine, Massage and Lymphatic Drainage massage from Nature Care College in Sydney. He is the author of *"Getting Healthy Naturally"* and has written many articles on the subject of health.

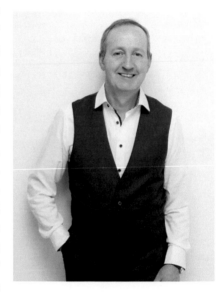

John lives in Navan, Co. Meath with his wife, Beulah, and their two young children, Shane and Olivia, and where he runs a busy natural healing centre for the past 20 years. You can visit him online at www.naturaltherapy.ie or phone his clinic at 046 9060702.

# Acknowledgements

My abundant and never-ending gratitude goes to my wife, Beulah Byrne.  Without her unconditional love, total support and undying belief in me, I would never have attempted to write this book.  She not only supports me in a myriad of personal ways but also gives me excellent editiorial input on every chapter.

To my 'organic' children Shane and Olivia; two special gifts straight from God and the most shining example of His grace in both Beulah's and my life.

And last but not least; to my clients, throughout the years – you are my inspiration and motivation to continue my healing ministry in the knowledge that I am helping people every day..... It's been an honour and a privilege to be a part of your care.

**John Byrne N.D., B.H.Sc.**

# Disclaimer and Waiver

## Note to the Reader

This book is intended as an educational tool to acquaint the reader with alternative methods of preventing and treating cancer. All the information I share in this book relating to natural medicine has been scientifically validated for years. I encourage you to take the time to review the hyperlinks and references that I have cited.

Because the methods described in this book are for the most part, considered alternative by definition, many of them have not been investigated or approved by governmental regulatory agencies. Accordingly, this book should not be substituted for the advice and medical treatment of an appropriately qualified specialist in the area of oncology.

Your health is important, use this book wisely. All the foods, remedies and supplements described in this book will work synergistically with your oncologist's programme. Your doctor should be made aware of any herbal medications and nutritional supplements you are taking. Search for a doctor who will support you with your goals of prevention or of healing.

Cancer therapy always carries a risk and the author or publisher cannot be in any way held responsible for outcome, adverse effects, lack of efficacy or other consequences that may happen as a result of using the information in this book. Ultimately, you the reader, must take full responsibility for your health and how you use this book.

# Contents

# INTRODUCTION

No one ever wants to hear the words, "I'm sorry but you have cancer," yet one in three will. It's one of the few words in the English language that can invoke fear and dread in the hearts and minds of anyone unfortunate enough to be given that diagnosis. Although trillions of dollars have been funnelled into cancer research to date, it still remains an undeterrable foe. Worldwide, the number of newly diagnosed cancer cases per year is expected to rise to 23.6 million by 2030.

Considering the trillions of dollars spent to stop this deadly scourge, the death rate from the most common cancers has not changed. About a third of all people who develop cancer still die from the disease, just as they did 50 years ago. The cancer patients who die of their disease are the ones who experience metastatic advanced spread of their tumours. Even with the most aggressive conventional treatments, only 5 to 10 percent of these patients will survive long term. For the other 90 to 95 percent, the gruelling enormously expensive treatment will add no more than a few months to their lives. In fact, there's evidence that those undergoing radical cancer treatment actually die sooner.

Even when cancers do appear to respond, these conventional treatments often erode away the patients own immune defences and end up doing more damage than good, or serve only as a temporary slowdown, leaving the door open for recurrence down the road.

But cash continues to pad the pockets of the pharmaceutical

companies. The consensus is that they are our saviour. That the cure will appear in synthetic form – without any side effects. It hasn't happened yet, nor will it! The truth is, there are many factors involved in the development of cancer, and equally there needs to be a multifactorial approach in its treatment, one that includes sound nutritional advice and guidance for fighting it. As you read through the pages of this book you'll come to realise why there aren't any one-shot wonder cures to be found. Instead, I champion a rich and varied approach, drawing on the best nature and medicine has to offer for the best outcomes imaginable.

One of the frustrations I often hear from my cancer clients is that their oncologists and family doctors are unfamiliar with nutritional therapies to prevent, treat and reduce recurrence of cancer. The only nutritional advice they get from their oncologist is to eat what they want so they can keep their weight up. Some even tell patients there's no relationship between their diet and cancer. The truth is your diet can make all the difference between recovering or succumbing to this nasty disease.

When my cancer clients mention the use of natural therapies to their oncologists to help fortify their natural defences against cancer, their physicians not only seem disinterested in the use of such therapies, no matter the evidence demonstrating their effectiveness, but some are downright hostile, believing that natural treatments will interfere with conventional treatments or have no benefit. Nothing could be further from the truth.

As you read through the pages of this book, you will gain a better understanding of cancer's modus operandi and how by using the natural approaches outlined herein, you can attack the disease via many methods by utilizing the biochemical peculiarities of the cancerous tumour against itself. So if you are fighting cancer now, I wish you success in your struggle and I hope that this book will contribute to your knowledge and lift your spirits. I know that cancer is a formidable foe, but in the course of my career as a naturopath I have known individuals with advanced cancers who have turned the tide in the most unpromising of situations. By following the scientifically-based and sound nutritional protocols outlined in this book along with my many other useful suggestions, these treatments helped put them on a path towards wellness. Some patients have gone into remission with nutritional and holistic therapies. Not only that, they have remained cancer free for many years.

---

**CHAPTER 1**

---

# What is Cancer?

*Cancer is a word, not a 'sentence'*– John Diamon

Scientists estimate that the human body is made up of approximately 37.2 trillion cells.[1] These cells grow and die every day. It is estimated that you lose five million cells every second to be replaced by another five million healthy daughter cells.

Each cell has its own particular function, for instance, a liver cell can only perform functions ascribed to the liver; a muscle cell won't suddenly become a bone cell.

Most body cells that have a purpose for developing, grow to their desired size and space out evenly in their tissue matrix, only dividing to replace worn out or damaged cells as required.

Normal cells undergo a process called APOPTOSIS or programmed cell death, in which the cell undergoes a series of genetically controlled events, which result in the destruction of unwanted cells without disruption or inflammation to surrounding tissues. Apoptotic cells are recognised by phagocytes (immune cells) and removed before they

1

disintegrate. As a result, there is no tissue damage or induction of inflammation.

Apoptosis is an important method of cellular control and any disruption of this process leads to abnormal growth of cells.

When the normal regulatory mechanism of a cell no longer works, it becomes mutant and will start to divide rapidly and keep multiplying in an uncontrolled manner. Since such cells have escaped the normal controls on proliferation they can divide as often as once every twenty minutes and before long that single rogue cell will have developed into a lump of cancerous cells or tumour.

By the time the tumour is big enough to be felt or detected by scans, it may contain billions of cancer cells. These cells do not die like normal cells and they even develop mechanisms to prevent detection by the immune system.

## Properties of Cancer Cells

In days of yore, warlords would carefully study their enemy's fortifications for any weaknesses that could be exploited in their quest to conquer them. Unfortunately for mankind, these same "Game of Thrones" scenarios still continue to this day with ever more cunning and deadly outcomes!

In a similar manner in the war against cancer, the fundamental properties of cancer cells have been carefully studied to reveal many inherent weaknesses in their makeup, which can then be exploited through various conventional and alternative means to help beat this dreaded disease.

Here's what has been discovered so far:

- Cancers arise from a single cell which has undergone mutation. Mutations occur at the genetic (DNA) level and can involve:
    - Gene deletion
    - Gene amplification
    - Point mutations
    - Chromosomal rearrangements

- All of which leads to irreversible cellular changes. This gives the cell increased growth advantages and the ability to escape normal controls on cell proliferation.

- The initial mutation will rapidly divide (as often as once every 20 minutes) to produce genetically similar clones. In other words this means that tumour suppressor genes within the cancer cell have failed.

- Additional mutations occur that further enhance the cells growth potential and create sub-clones within the tumour mass with certain dangerous propensities (e.g. cancer stems cells, which are a type of "seed" cell that can literally pump out millions of daughter cells that form tumours).

- Cancer stem cells can synthesize a special protein on their outer membrane that shields or cloaks them from the immune system.

- Cancer stem cells can metastasize, meaning they can spread to another part of the body via the blood stream or lymphatic system, forming secondary cancers.

- Cancer cells can produce a protein called *"survivin"* which prevents the cancer cell from going through the natural cycle of death, known as "Apoptosis" or programmed cell death.

- Cancer cells are "Anchorage independent" meaning they do not require contact with the surface of other cells or tissues in order to grow unlike normal cells.

- Cancer cells are less adhesive than normal cells and so, can spread more easily throughout the body.

- Cancer cells are not sensitive to cell density (unlike normal cells) in their proliferation and so, invade neighbouring tissues and organs.

- For a cancer tumour to survive and thrive there needs to be inflammation in the surrounding tissues. This inflammation can be generated via the cancer cell's metabolic processes and also be present as a result of an "inverted way" of living such as poor dietary and lifestyle choices. In my book, *"Getting Healthy*

*Naturally"* I delve into the topic of inflammation and how it can be generated via a myriad of ways. In the book I explain in great detail how to quench this inflammation by addressing all the underlying factors that contribute to it, for example:

- Dietary factors
- Environmental toxins
- Infectious agents
- Digestive dysbiosis (poor gut health)
- Food sensitivities
- Lifestyle and psychological factors, such as no exercise or extreme exercise, poor sleep, mental and emotional stress, etc.
- Obesity
- Injuries that don't fully heal
- An overly acidic metabolism

- Cancer cells thrive best in an acidic environment (causes inflammation) so making the body more alkaline inhibits cancer growth.

- Cancer cells can actually create an acidic environment in the body by means of their cellular respiration. Let me explain the process, cellular respiration in cancer cells versus normal cells.

  Normal cells get their energy through a process called *"oxidative phosphorylation"* taking place in the mitochondria (powerhouse of the cell). These reactions produce ATP (energy for the cell), which is used by the cell to carry out their life-sustaining metabolic functions. This process involves taking in oxygen and glucose (a simple sugar) and the result is 32 molecules of ATP for every molecule of glucose metabolised.

  Cancer cells on the other hand do not use oxygen for generating energy (a fact discovered as far back as 1932 by Dr. Otto Warburg). In fact, cancer cells hate oxygen. They get their energy through a process called ANAEROBIC respiration (without oxygen), a very inefficient system that produces only two molecules of ATP for every molecule of glucose metabolised. This process generates high amounts of lactic acid as waste, the same substance that causes cramps in athletes. Lactic acid is very toxic and causes inflammation to surrounding tissues.

- Cancer is an "OBLIGATE GLUCOSE METABOLIZER" meaning that it thrives best on simple sugars like glucose. Because of their defective metabolism, cancer cells cannot convert complex carbohydrates, fats or proteins (with the exception of glutamine, an amino acid) into the energy currency ATP. The fact that these cells are such poor glucose metabolisers makes them so ravenous about having to continuously absorb sugar to survive. Hence, one of the ways to combat cancer is to reduce or eliminate sugar in your diet so as not to feed the cancer.

- Cancer cells have the ability to grow their own blood vessels in order to supply the tumour with a good supply of nutrition. This process is called *ANGIOGENESIS*. Restricting the growth of the tumour's blood vessels, either by using conventional agents or by using herbal or nutraceutical agents, is also an opportunity to help defeat cancer.

## WHAT CAUSES CANCER?

This is the million dollar question and there is no simple answer. Saying that, we know that cancer is a complex disease with many known causes. Over the past hundred years or so, many theories have been put forward to explain cancer initiation as well as the main triggers and predisposing factors that support the cancer process.

In the previous section I outlined the hallmarks of cancer which gives insight into the ways cancer needs to be addressed in its prevention and treatment. These hallmarks as agreed upon by the oncology community are neatly summarised in the following statement:

*The hallmarks of cancer comprise eight biological capabilities acquired by incipient cancer cells during the multistep development of human tumours. The hallmarks constitute an organising principle for rationalizing the complexities of neoplastic disease. They include:*

- *Sustaining proliferative signaling*
- *Evading growth suppressors*
- *Resisting cell death*
- *Enabling replicative immortality*
- *Inducing angiogenesis*
- *Activating invasion and metastasis*
- *Reprogramming energy metabolism*
- *Evading immune destruction* (2)

The authors further state that *"facilitating the acquisition of these hallmark capabilities are genome instability, which enables mutational alteration of hallmark-enabling genes and immune inflammation, which fosters the acquisition of multiple hallmark functions."*(2) In other words, the official position as adopted by all major cancer institutions is that cancer is purely a genetic disease whereupon certain genetic changes alter the way cells divide, resulting in various mutations and tumour growths.

Let's examine this theory along with other theories that have been proposed regarding the initiation of the cancer process.

# THEORY ONE:
# THE GENETIC THEORY

This is the predominant theory of the orthodox oncology community, namely that cancer occurs due to changes in the genes responsible for cell growth and repair. As a result, all the descendants of that aberrant cell will contain its altered DNA and these cells form tumours.(3) Among the classes of genes in a human cell is a group called cancer genes which are broadly grouped into "Oncogenes" (that promote cancer growth) and "Tumour Suppressor" genes (that halt cancer growth). If a mutation occurs in either of these gene types, the cell is likely to mutate to a cancer cell.

Also, any faulty genes that were passed down to us by our parents and grandparents can be major determining factors in whether or not we as individuals will develop cancer at some point in our lives. For example, the BRCA1 and BRCA2 genes can lead to the development of breast and ovarian cancer. The APC gene may be responsible for a number of cancers. About 25% of prostate cancers are believed to be inherited and may be caused by a mutation of the HPC1, HPC2, HPCX, or CAPB gene. Mutations in any of these genes mean they are unable to repair damaged DNA, leading to a higher risk of cancer. Individuals who have these inherited genes need to be extremely careful in their diet, lifestyle and environment so that they don't activate these genes in the first place.

Certain lifestyle and environmental factors such as chemical exposure and radiation can change normal genes into faulty ones that facilitate cancer growth. Risk factors that adversely influence cellular DNA include:

- Smoking
- Poor diet
- High alcohol consumption
- Exposure to carcinogens
- Excessive sunlight as well as other types of radiation
- Ageing

The important thing to consider for now is the control of those things that cause or fuel cancer via genetic means (carcinogens, etc.) by either avoiding them or mitigating them.

# THEORY TWO:
# CHROMOSOMAL INSTABILITY

Healthy human cells have 23 different pairs of chromosomes, which add up to a total of 46 individual chromosomes in somatic cells. Cancer cells, on the other hand typically have between 60 to 90 individual chromosomes. Now according to Davis Rasnick PhD, an independent researcher in oncogenesis, cancer cells always display the characteristics of chromosomal instability, a defect that involves loss or rearrangement of the cells genetic material, i.e. chromosomes during cell division (called mitosis). These severely damaged chromosomes result in the duplication or loss of thousands of genes and this type of process is referred to as "ANEUPLOIDY". [4] This chromosome trait is unique to cancer cells, as normal cells in the body strictly maintain the correct number and structure of chromosomes.

Recall that genes are individual units that are strung along the chromosomes so that each chromosome contains thousands of genes (approximately 20,000 genes in each human cell). Any cell with a chromosome number different from 46 will have a different complement of genes and chromosomes compared to a normal cell. This imbalance leads to a variety of health problems, one of which is cancer.

One well-known example of an imbalanced chromosome number is Down's syndrome. This results when a baby is born with three copies of chromosome 21 instead of the normal two. Just one extra copy of this smaller chromosome is sufficient to cause this syndrome.

In the case of Down's syndrome the chromosomal defect occurs in the sex chromosomes (germ cells) and so, the chromosomal error is present in every cell in the body. In the case of cancer, the defects that give rise to the unbalanced complement of chromosomes occur in the somatic cells (individual body cells).

Somatic cells constantly divide to produce identical daughter cells by a process called *Mitosis*. When errors in mitosis occur, as they often do, aberrant cells will result. When these aberrant daughter cells continue to divide, their genetic material becomes increasingly disorganised to the point where most of these cells stop dividing and die. However, if advantages conferred by the changes in chromosome copy number are somehow capable of overcoming apoptosis (programmed cell death) then these aberrant cells become cancer cells and cancer formation is most likely.

The chromosomal instability theory of cancer was first introduced by David Von Hansemann in 1890 *(5)* and expounded upon by Theodor Boveri in 1914.*(6)* One of the first things that both researchers noticed when they observed cancer cells under the microscope was that they had excess chromosomes. Boveri hypothesized that cancer results from a certain abnormal constitution, the way in which it originates having no significance. Each process (i.e. cell division), which brings about this constitution would result in the origin of a malignant tumour. *(6)* In other words his theory predicts that cancer results from a single cell that has acquired an abnormal chromosome constitution.

One ardent believer in the chromosomal instability theory of cancer (as opposed to the genetic mutation theory) is Dr David Rasnick of UC, Berkeley who has demonstrated that in order to transform a normal cell into a cancer cell, massive changes are required in the number and composition of chromosomes and not just a few gene mutations *(7)*.

Dr Rasnick, a former mainstream researcher who has now become an outsider, presents an explanation of cancer by tracing the cause to chromosome malfunction, which is a major departure from the orthodox view of cancer being gene mutation.

In his hypothesis, Rasnick claims:

1. The biggest mark against the gene mutation hypothesis is that every attempt to experimentally, or any other way, to prove it has failed.
2. Basing diagnostic and subsequent treatment on the gene theory has failed to reduce the incidence of cancer and mortality. When you think about it, the major focus of research has been based on the genetic theory for over 50 years and now with the mapping of the human genome complete, this has not led to any significant cancer "cures" as originally thought.

3. Theoretical and experimental proof that unbalanced chromosomes cause cancer continues to amass. *(8)* Dr Rasnick also claims with proof, that "the scrambling of chromosomes is so massive that no two cancer cells are identical." *(8)*

# THEORY THREE:
# TROPHOBLAST THEORY OF CANCER

Dr John Beard (1857 - 1924) a British embryologist and histologist first proposed his trophoblast theory of cancer in 1902, which states that certain pre-embryonic cells (called trophoblasts) in pregnancy differ in no discernible way from highly malignant cancer cells. *(9)*

He devised his theory after observing a link between the development of cancer in an unborn foetus shortly after day 56 of pregnancy and the abnormal development of the foetal pancreas. This was the key to Beard's discovery of the link between cancer and pancreatic insufficiency - that cancer is actually the result of fast-growing trophoblast cells that the body failed to terminate through pancreatic secretions.

Trophoblasts are specialised cells of the placenta formed during the first stage of pregnancy. These cells act and behave in a manner identical to cancer cells, multiplying and spreading rapidly as they eat their way into the uterine lining to prepare a nest for the embryo to attach itself for nourishment and protection.

Dr. Beard observed that on day 56 of gestation, trophoblast cells transform from their malignant invasive nature into stable cells of the placenta. He noticed that day 56 also coincided with the appearance of pancreatic enzymes when the foetal pancreas fully forms.

It was well known then that the developing foetus obtains all its nutrition from the mother's blood supply and so has no need for pancreatic enzymes to digest its food at this stage of development. Beard theorised that there must be another reason for these enzymes to appear so early in the pregnancy, and he came up with the explanation that they were responsible for terminating trophoblast activity. He reasoned that these pancreatic enzymes eat through the outer layer of any trophoblast cells they encounter, digesting any markers that identify them as host cells, and so making them vulnerable to destruction by the immune system.

Beard further theorised that cancer, while having multifactorial triggers that will initiate uncontrolled trophoblast activity, has in fact one root cause, and that is a deficiency of pancreatic enzymes. He maintained that trophoblasts left over from embryonic development of the foetus are scattered throughout our bodies and later in life, can be stimulated by what we would call an initiator or carcinogen to begin reproducing, or give rise to a kind of embryo in the wrong time and wrong place. He contends that it is the job of the pancreas with its pancreatic enzymes to digest those leftover trophoblast cells the moment they begin to multiply. If there is a deficiency of pancreatic enzymes, these primitive undifferentiated cells begin to multiply and the result is cancer. Beard subsequently suggested the supplementation of pancreatic enzymes to control cancer.

Beard's model of cancer has subsequently been expanded in the 1960s by William D. Kelley (1926-2005) who had considerable success treating cancer patients with pancreatic enzyme therapy and in more recent times by the late Dr Nicholas Gonzalez of New York. *(10)*

Modern advances in our understanding of molecular and cell biology, especially in the area of stem cell research have found remarkable similarities between trophoblasts and cancer cells. They have both been shown to have similar molecular mechanisms for their proliferative, invasive and metastatic capacities.

We now know that trophoblast cells originate from another type of cell called stem cells. Stem cells have the capacity to evolve into any tissue, organ or embryo. They exist all over the body and their purpose is to initiate repair and growth of damaged tissue. In Dr Beard's day he wouldn't have known the true purpose of stem cells outside the reproductive organs, and so he speculated that they were escaped cells left over from embryogenesis.

It's now known that if stem cells come into contact with the hormone oestrogen (present in both females and males) they transform into trophoblast cells. At this stage one of two things can happen:

- In the case of pregnancy, the result of the development of the placenta to assist embryo growth or
- As part of the healing process to repair damaged tissue.

It is interesting to note that if tissue is taken from a wound that is undergoing repair and examined under a microscope, the histopathologist would not be able to differentiate it from a cancerous tumour. *(11)* So when you think about it, a wound undergoing healing is actually cancerous in nature, or to be more accurate, we should say it is cancer if the healing process is not terminated upon completion of its task! Some cancer researchers refer to cancer as the *"wound that never heals."* In fact, it is not uncommon for someone to develop cancer following a major operation or injury such as a broken hip or leg.

## The Hormone Connection

Trophoblast cells release their own hormone called human chorionic gonadotropin (HCG). The detection of this hormone is the basis for the common pregnancy test. Because cancer cells are like trophoblast cells then it stands to reason that one would expect cancer cells to also produce HCG hormones.

In 1995 such evidence was provided by Professor Hernan Acevedo and colleagues and was published in The Journal of Cancer. *(12)* They found that every type of cancer produces HCG hormone, similar to the trophoblast cells of pregnancy. In his 1995 report Dr Acevedo concluded that after nearly a century, Beard has been proven to be conceptually correct.

# THEORY FOUR:
# STEM CELL THEORY

This theory can stake its origin from Beard's trophoblast theory of cancer. According to our present knowledge of stem cell research, stem cells exist all over the body having been deposited there during the process of embryogenesis. Beard thought that stem cells were germ cells (i.e. sex cells that can only produce a baby) that somehow escaped normal controls and lay dormant in body tissues until some initiator or insult stimulated them into action whereupon they become cancerous.

What Beard didn't know at the time was that the purpose of stem cells is to initiate the repair and regrowth of damaged tissues and organs and those stem cells are endowed with the ability to reproduce themselves and change into any type of body cell depending on the tissue or organ they are situated in.

Stem cells remain dormant in all body tissues and organs until called upon to repair damaged tissue. During the repair process there is a great deal of inflammation taking place (think of the heat, redness and swelling that occurs if you bruise your finger), as a result of the cascade of inflammatory mediators being released by immune cells as part of the repair process. This inflammatory process generates intense storms of free radicals and lipid peroxidation products that can damage the DNA of stem cells.

Based on the observation that stem cells are as vulnerable to free radical damage as ordinary cells in the body are, it is proposed that cancerous tumours originate from mutated stem cells that somehow had their DNA damaged. (13) These mutated stem cells become rogue, reproducing themselves in mass numbers to sustain the cancer. In essence, these damaged stem cells generate the developing cancer, much like normal stem cells renew and sustain our organs and tissues.

The cancer cells being produced by the mutated stem cells resemble, in a crude way, the cells found in normal tissue. However, these daughter cells cannot reproduce themselves; it is only the stem cells that can reproduce.

An easy way to understand this theory of cancer development is to visualise the mutated cancer stem cell like a child's bubble blower making bubbles. The film of soap on the ring of the bubble blower can be compared to the cancer stem cell and the steady stream of bubbles emanating from the ring are the newly formed cancer cells.

These new cancer cells that are being produced form the bulk of the tumour and unlike the cancer stem cells, which produced them, they cannot divide or reproduce. *(13)* In cancer studies, researchers now know that cancer stem cells are essential for tumour growth and that the tumour mass consists of only 1% of cancer stem cells. *(14)*

When treating a person who has cancer, unless you kill the mutated cancer stem cell population, or somehow convert them back to normal stem cells, the cancer will continue to recur. Conventional cancer treatments such as chemotherapy and radiation can easily shrink tumours by killing the daughter cells being produced by the cancer stem cells; however, studies show that cancer stem cells are highly resistant to these treatments. If these therapies are not killing the cancer stem cells, the tumour will soon grow back and in the process, become even more virulent and resistant to these toxic treatments. That's usually when the patient is told that they are not responding to their treatment anymore, and that there's nothing further that can be done other than to get their affairs in order. However, various studies that I will refer to in this book suggest that there are several natural substances that can either kill cancer stem cells or convert them back to normal stem cells.

# THEORY FIVE:
## OTTO WARBURG'S THEORY OF DAMAGED CELLULAR RESPIRATION

Dr Otto Warburg (1883-1971) won the Nobel Prize in medicine in 1931 for his discovery of the oxygen-transferring enzyme of cellular respiration. *(15)* What this means is that he discovered the mechanism by which oxygen is transported in and out of the cells. This work led him into the study of cancer, specifically cancer cell metabolism, whereupon he discovered that cancer cells were low in oxygen due to a change in the way in which they generated their energy needs.

Warburg's theory is based around the fact that human cells have two ways of generating energy. The first type of energy production is called "Aerobic" respiration, where the cell uses oxygen to oxidize or burn sugars. This is a very efficient method of obtaining maximum energy per molecule of glucose for cellular use (known as ATP or Adenosine triphosphate). For aerobic respiration to correctly work, the cells oxygen-transferring enzymes that transfer oxygen from outside to inside the cell must be fully functioning, and also, there needs to be sufficient oxygen available in the bloodstream.

If normal healthy cells cannot obtain sufficient oxygen from the bloodstream to keep aerobic respiration going, cells will then switch over to another method of generating their energy needs without the use of oxygen.

This second energy-producing process is called "ANAEROBIC" respiration and it basically involves glucose being fermented into lactic acid. This is a very inefficient energy producing system that produces only two modules of ATP per glucose module metabolised compared to the 38 modules of ATP produced by aerobic respiration.

Warburg postulated that cancer arises from a cell trying to perform all its normal functions on the limited energy supply generated from anaerobic (fermentation) respiration. In order for the cell to survive and thrive using only fermentation as an energy source, the cell will change back (mutate) to a more primitive form, where it lacks the control that limits cell division and proliferation. Warburg likens this transition from aerobic respiration to anaerobic respiration as a transition from "heaven to hell". (16) In his own words Warburg says that *"cancer above all other diseases has countless secondary causes. But, even for cancer, there is only one prime cause. Summarised in a few words, the prime cause of cancer is the replacement of the respiration of oxygen in normal body cells by a fermentation of sugar."* (17)

To prove his theory he devised a simple experiment using cultured cells in an oxygen-controlled environment and demonstrated that when the oxygen supply was reduced by 35% of the cells requirement for a period of 48 hours, the ensuing daughter cells started to manifest cancer cells properties.

This led him to hypothesize that oxygen might be used to cure cancer. However when he tested his hypothesis and tried to cure cancer with oxygen, he failed. He later came to realise that the cancer process is multifactorial and the factors that bring about damaged cellular respiration in cancer cells can be listed under three categories:

1. Respiratory poisons, in our food, air and water (i.e. smoke, chemicals, pesticides, exhaust fumes, food additives, etc.)
2. Insufficient oxygen supply to cells for a prolonged period.
3. Cellular strain caused by neighbouring cells that have switched over to fermentation thereby creating an acidic environment.

Warburg proposed the following recommendations for ensuring we do not get cancer and as a therapeutic approach in the treatment of cancer:

- Cleaning our environment and body of all respiratory poisons (carcinogenic toxins).
- Dietary supplementation with vitamins and minerals known to enhance cellular respiration.
- Exercise to enhance blood flow and ensure adequate oxygenation of body tissues and cells.
- Use of therapies that increase oxygenation within the body so as to increase aerobic respiration within cells (i.e. hyperbaric oxygen chambers, ozone therapy)

These recommendations are geared towards doing everything possible to clean up our body's unhealthy cellular terrain and create an environment conducive to efficient cellular (aerobic) respiration.

# THEORY SIX:
# THE METABOLIC ORIGIN OF CANCER

Expanding upon Warburg's theory of damaged cellular respiration, we now know that impaired cellular energy metabolism is the defining characteristic of nearly all cancers regardless of cellular or tissue origin.

To recap briefly: Warburg's observation was that: cancer cells have a perverted method of generating energy. They curtail the conversion of glucose into energy. They depend much less on the efficient process of aerobic respiration, using oxygen to produce energy, instead relying much more on the ancient and highly inefficient pathway known as fermentation.

Following his extensive research on cancer metabolism, Warburg stated: *"cancer, above all other diseases, has countless secondary causes. But, even for cancer there is only one prime cause. Summarised in a few words, the prime cause of cancer is the replacement of the respiration of oxygen in normal body cells by a fermentation of sugar."* *(17)*

Expanding upon Warburg's hypothesis, Boston College Biology Professor, Dr Thomas N. Seyfried and author of the book "Cancer as a Metabolic Disease", noted that, across the board, all cancer cells have damaged cellular organelles called mitochondria. Typically, each healthy cell in the body contains between 1,000 and 2,000 mitochondria. Mitochondria are thought of as the cellular power plants. They generate energy through oxidative respiration (using oxygen) supplying the body with the energy it needs to function. The damaged mitochondria unable to generate enough energy for cellular survival then send out emergency signals to the cell's nucleus for it to switch on emergency measures. When the cell's DNA responds, the entire complexion of the cell changes. It begins to exhibit the hallmark features of cancer, namely, gene mutation and/or chromosomal abnormality, uncontrolled cellular replication, evasion of programmed natural cell death (apoptosis), and so forth.

So, in a nutshell, the cell's nuclear genetic defects, typically thought to be responsible for cancer actually occur further downstream. Mitochondrial damage happens first, which then triggers genetic and chromosomal mutations that may lead to cancer. *(18)*

Seyfried contends that Warburg's idea on the primary cause of cancer, i.e., the replacement of oxidative respiration by fermentation, was only a symptom of cancer and not the cause. Ongoing research now questions the genetic origin of cancer, still held in high esteem by the scientific bedrock of institutional cancer research and suggests that cancer is primarily a metabolic disease.

In the introduction to his recently released book (2017) *"Tripping Over The Truth - how the Metabolic Theory of Cancer is overturning one of medicine's most entrenched paradigms,"* author Travis Christofferson teases the reader with the proposition:

*"Maybe we've mischaracterized the origin of cancer. Maybe cancer is not a genetic disease after all. Maybe we are losing the war against cancer, because scientists are chasing a flawed scientific paradigm, and cancer is not a disease of damaged DNA, but rather one of defective metabolism."*

So, if cancer is primarily a disease of defective energy metabolism, then rational approaches to cancer treatment can be found in therapies that specifically target energy metabolism. The good news is that you can optimise your mitochondrial function by addressing certain lifestyle factors such as diet and exercise, and this knowledge opens up a whole new way of looking at and treating cancer.


# THEORY SEVEN:
# PLEOMORPHISM AND THE CANCER MICROBE

For more than 100 years there is increasing evidence for a microbial cause of cancer. For example, the distinguished pathologist William Russell (1852-1940) in 1890 discovered that there are microbes inside and outside of cancer cells. *(19)*

Throughout the intervening years several other independent

researchers have also reported the proliferation of certain microbes in all cancer patients. One of the first was Dr Gunther Enderlein, a German professor of microbiology and zoology who described in 1925 the different stages of a microbe that is normally present in the blood as tiny colloidal particles, which he named 'protits'. He found that these tiny protein-based microorganisms flourished in the blood and cells in a mutually beneficial relationship with their host. However, any deterioration in the hosts internal environment could cause these protits to change from innocuous agents into viruses, then into increasingly higher bacterial forms and finally into fungi. Each of these stages is progressively more hostile to surrounding tissue. These altered forms are referred to as "pleomorphic", that is, they change shape and size depending on the level of toxicity of the host's tissue. [20]

## PLEOMORPHISM: Its discovery and repression

Back in the 1870s when Louis Pasteur (1822-1895) went public with his 'germ theory' of disease, a French physician and pharmacist Antoine Béchamp (1816-1908), a much more qualified and experienced researcher, was also looking at the new frontier world of microbes. He came up with a more complex but thorough understanding of these miniature marvels.

Béchamp identified a fundamental unit of microbiological life, which he claimed was critical in supporting the life of cells. He named this unit **microzyma**. [21] Béchamp declared that these microzyma can change shape (morph) and in fact, take on many sequential shapes (pleo) that are increasingly pathogenic depending on specific changes in the state of the hosts internal environment.

Béchamp showed the germs actually originated from inside the body from tiny dots that change form and shape into microorganisms that clean up the toxins, garbage and dead cells that are the result of toxic conditions within the body.

These pleomorphic microorganisms that Pasteur observed through his microscope, i.e., the viruses, bacteria and fungi, which he blamed as the cause of the disease, were observed by Béchamp as being part of nature's "cleanup crew", breaking down sick tissue and ultimately decomposing it.

Béchamp coined the term *pleomorphism,* which refers to the ability of microbes to change from one form into another; from a seed (microzyma) to a virus, to a bacteria and finally into fungal states, rather than being seen as discrete species unto themselves. Once these microbes have done their clean-up job they revert back to their seed stage once again ready to support new life.

However, the Germ Theory of Louis Pasteur was fully embraced by the scientific establishment of the day, who were looking for a simple and straightforward explanation of disease. Even to this day conventional science still subscribes to the concept of "monomorphism", the notion that microbes always maintain their basic shape as virus, bacterium or fungus, and cannot change from one form to another.

This simplistic notion of "kill the bug" cure of disease that's embraced by the pharmaceutical industry is akin to trying to get rid of flies; while it would make more sense to clean up the garbage attracting them in the first place. Now of course infectious agents may enter the body from outside, but if the body is healthy and its cellular terrain balanced, these agents will not thrive or even survive.

Other research pioneers, mostly without knowing of each other's work, corroborated Béchamp's pleomorphic theory. One such researcher was French biologist Gaston Naessens, who developed an optic microscope that allowed him to view living organisms at high magnification. With this tool, he saw tiny particles in the blood, which he named "somatids" [22] similar to the microzyma of Béchamp, or the protit of Enderlein.

Naessen discovered that somatids go through a 3-stage life cycle when the body is healthy. These are non pathogenic states. However, if the body's internal environment becomes stressed or toxic, these somatids evolve through a macrocycle of 13 additional states, becoming ever more pathogenic. [23] Many of these new states have been associated with different diseases including cancer.

# Royal Raymond Rife

Several other research scientists have independently identified pleomorphic microbes as being the fundamental cause of cancer. Chief among them was Dr Royal Raymond Rife (1888 - 1971), a microbiologist who in the 1930s proved that if the microbes inside the cancer cells are destroyed, the cancer cells will revert back to normal cells.

Rife was also a brilliant technician who developed a microscope, which gave resolutions up to 50,000 times compared to 2,000 resolutions of the day. With his "universal microscope" as he termed it, Rife was able to observe and prove the fact of pleomorphism. Due to his knowledge of optics and because he used light frequencies to highlight his samples rather than chemical dyes (which kill microbes) his microscope was the only one that was able to view live viruses and other living microbes.

When he studied blood samples of cancer patients, Rife saw the same tiny virus-sized organisms in all of his cancer patients. He named this microbe "Bacillus X or BX, and when he injected this microbe into healthy mice, all of them developed cancer.

Dr Rife also developed a machine called the Rife Frequency Generator. His machine was designed to do one thing, kill microbes. Rife discovered that if you play an harmonic electromagnetic frequency to a microorganism, it will oscillate or vibrate with the frequency until it literally bursts; much like the way an opera singer can shatter a crystal glass with the right singing pitch.

So with his universal microscope, Rife was able to isolate the particular viral form involved in all types of cancer and by using his frequency generator discovered an harmonic resonant frequency to vibrate the cancer microbes until they shattered and died. His frequency generator was not designed to kill cancer cells but only to kill the microbes inside the cancer cells as well as similar microbes in the blood and in the interstitial spaces between cells. When all the microbes are destroyed, the cancer cells will revert back to normal cells. Many people were subsequently cured of cancer with his device during the 1930s.

Indeed the possibilities of this revolutionary machine sent shockwaves through the cancer industry when Dr Milbank Johnson conducted a study of the Rife Frequency Generator as a potential cancer treatment. Dr Johnson coordinated the study with the Medical Research Committee of the University of Southern California in 1934.

Sixteen patients with various types of advanced cancer, all of whom had been declared terminal or incurable, were included in the study. Their treatment protocol involved the use of the Rife Frequency Generator for daily treatments of 3 minutes duration, at 3-day intervals. After 3 months of the Rife treatments, 14 of these incurable cases were declared clinically cured and in good health by a staff of 5 doctors and also by Dr Alvin G. Ford, group pathologist. The other two subsequently recovered full health shortly after the end of the trial. In other words a 100% cure rate on patients in the worst possible condition. *(24)*

Rife should have won the Nobel Prize in medicine for his discovery of the cause and cure for cancer, but unfortunately the Cancer Industry in cahoots with the Food and Drug Administration (FDA) and the American Medical Association (AMA) sought to discredit Dr Rife and his Rife Frequency Generator.

You may ask why? Well it all comes down to money; a guy called Maurice Fishbien who at the time was Head Editor of the journal of the AMA, wanted to buy into Rife's discovery for personal gain. When Rife rejected this request, Fishbien used his position to maliciously vilify Rife and his discoveries and together with the FDA, they outlawed the Rife Frequency Generator as a treatment for cancer. The sad fact is that the FDA, the AMA and the Cancer Industry in general, have little or no desire to cure cancer, because treating cancer as a chronic disease is thousands of times more profitable than curing it!!

# How do Microbes turn cells cancerous?

The cancer microbe is highly pleomorphic and has been observed to literally drill its way through the cell wall of a healthy cell and turn it into a cancer cell.

Scientists from the Independent Cancer Research Foundation (ICRF), a non-profit foundation, investigating natural cancer treatments discovered how cancer microbes inside cells produce toxic metabolites that block the oxidative energy production of the affected cells.

Here is the chain of events that turns normal cells cancerous, as proposed by the ICRF researchers; (25)

- Once inside a cell, the microbe intercepts the glucose entering the cell (most microbes eat glucose)
- The microbe excretes toxic metabolites called "mycotoxins" as waste.
- Because mycotoxins are highly acidic, the inside of the cell becomes very acidic (acidity is a characteristic of cancer cells).
- The cells mitochondria, which convert glucose into ATP (energy), get very little glucose because the microbe has intercepted most of the glucose.
- As a result, cellular energy levels plummet as the mitochondria are bathed in an increasingly large sea of mycotoxins.
- More signals are sent to the glucose receptors on the cell membrane (wall) to grab more glucose.
- More glucose floods into the cell (up to 15 times more than normal) but most of the glucose is intercepted by the rapidly dividing microbes.
- These microbes also create a thick protein coating on the outside of the cell wall which attracts more glucose, but also blocks oxygen from entering the cell (microbes hate oxygen).
- The cells mitochondria already bathed in a sea of highly acidic mycotoxins, now have to contend with a shortage of

oxygen, and so, the cell is forced to derive its energy by using anaerobic (fermentation) respiration.

- This causes the cell to become even more acidic, and as we already know from the research of Otto Warburg that the defining characteristic of cancer cells is low ATP energy output as a result of fermentation, it can now be stated that the cell is cancerous.

So the above hypothesis explaining how microbes can cause cancer is very plausible and has many facts to back it up. In fact, David J. Hess, a professor in the Sociology Department at Vanderbilt University, Nashville wrote a fascinating book linking microbes as the underlying cause of many cancers. [26]

It is now known that many cancers can originate from infectious organisms (i.e. viruses, bacteria, fungi).

**For example:**

- Human Papilloma virus (HPV) is associated with at least 80% of all cervical cancer.
- Helicobacter Pylori, the bacteria that causes stomach ulcers is also a major risk factor for stomach cancer.
- The Epstein-Barr virus that causes glandular fever is also a known cause of Burkitt's lymphoma, a type of cancer of the lymphatic system.
- Chronic infection with hepatitis B and C viruses can cause liver cancer.
- Aflatoxins are toxic compounds produced by certain fungi (often affecting peanuts) which can also cause liver cancer when ingested excessively.

Dr. Tullio Simoncina, an Italian oncologist who wrote an interesting book, "Cancer is a Fungus," believes that cancer is mainly due to Candida Albicans, the most common and aggressive fungus in the human body. His research reveals that cancer cells and candida yeast cells have a similar fermentation (energy) metabolism. As a consequence of toxic overload building up in the body, candida spores can change into more aggressive and invasive hyphal forms that look like and behave in the same way as cancer cells.

Simoncina believes that cancer is a fungus that will do what all fungi do – form colonies and spread throughout the host area. His cure is to alkalise the body to produce conditions in which the candida cannot thrive. Part of his treatment protocol includes the use of Sodium Bicarbonate (baking soda) to change the pH of the cancer tumour from one of acidity (which cancer cells love) to alkalinity.

Simoncina's assertion that all types of cancer originate from candida albicans, and can therefore be treated with a simple compound like sodium bicarbonate, in my opinion, is simplistic reasoning for this complex and multifactorial disease that has its roots at the cellular level. With cancer we are in essence dealing with a chronic metabolic disease that cries out for a holistic response, to include fundamental changes in our diet and lifestyle. When the body's internal environment becomes toxic and out of balance, pleomorphic microbes increasingly block aerobic energy metabolism of affected cells forcing them to start producing energy anaerobically, similar to fungi like candida albicans. When this happens cancer cells begin to act and look like fungal cells.

However, the aerobic energy metabolism of cancer cells can be fully restored, converting them back to healthy non-cancerous cells by eliminating the cancer-causing microbes and their toxins that block aerobic respiration. This cannot be done with candida. This fungus will always produce its energy by fermentation.

# OTHER CONTRIBUTING FACTORS TO CANCER DEVELOPMENT

## POOR IMMUNE FUNCTION

Your immune system is your major defence against foreign invaders such as viruses, bacteria, fungi and parasites. Its job is to detect these unwelcome organisms and swiftly destroy and eliminate them before they can do any real harm.

Likewise, it should also protect you from cancer cells. It should recognise them as being foreign and kill them. This is what a healthy immune system does. Yet, clearly if you have cancer, your immune system has somehow failed. It could be argued therefore, that cancer is primarily a problem with the immune system.

Everyday we develop cancer cells throughout our bodies. Our immune cells are normally able to find them, identify them and destroy them before they are able to grow uncontrollably. It is a normal occurrence, which is constantly taking place in a healthy body. It is only when a weakened immune system becomes unable to mount its normal defence that cancer cells can escape to proliferate and spread uncontrollably.

So cancer cannot develop if you have a fully functioning immune system. If you do have cancer, you don't have an intact immune system, it is somehow compromised. Therefore, in the treatment of cancer it is vital to figure out the underlying root causes of this immune failure and address these causes appropriately.

As a matter of interest, if you do have cancer, it is not entirely the fault of your immune system, because cancer cells have developed some very clever ways of hiding from it and avoiding attack by it. They can secrete specific enzymes to put the immune system to sleep, or to switch off the immune system's identifying capabilities. Nonetheless a healthy immune system is vitally important as your protector in the fight against cancer.

## CHRONIC INFLAMMATION (The common link in all cancers)

If there is a defining truth about the etiology of cancer that is beyond argument, it is that cancer has multiple interacting causes. Factors such as microbial infections, genetic abnormalities, low cellular oxygen, environmental carcinogens, toxic overload and a dysfunctional immune system are some of the factors already discussed that contribute to the development of cancer.

However, there is one central factor most closely associated with cancer development and that is "conventional cancer treatments,"[27] In the first book I wrote called, *"Getting Healthy Naturally"* I explained in great detail the role that chronic inflammation plays in the etiology of all diseases including cancer.

Various studies have been carried out on groups of people who have cancer and compared with people who never had cancer. What the researchers discovered is that the people who developed cancer, in most cases had previously suffered from some sort of inflammatory disease such as arthritis, an autoimmune condition, or an underlying chronic infection that preceded the cancer diagnosis by between 10 and 17 years. These same researchers also noticed that the longer the inflammation persists, the higher the risk of developing cancer.

There is now a substantial body of evidence to support the conclusion that chronic inflammation can predispose an individual to cancer, as demonstrated by the association between well known inflammatory bowel diseases such as crohn's disease and ulcerative colitis, and a corresponding higher incidence of bowel cancer in these individuals when compared to the general population.

Many other cancers are known to arise from sites of infection, chronic irritation and inflammation. In general, the longer the inflammation persists the higher the risk of developing cancer.

The most widely studied and best established of these links are colon cancer associated with inflammatory bowel disease; chronic helicobacter pylori infection of the stomach as a precursor to stomach cancer; Hepatitis B and C virus associated with liver cancer; Human papillomavirus (HPV), Herpes virus and Cytomegalovirus are all implicated in cervical, ovarian and other cancers.

Another well-known inflammation-induced cancer is lung cancer, caused either by cigarette smoke or asbestos that both initiate chronic inflammation in the airways, leading to a higher incidence of lung cancer in these individuals.

## THE GOOD AND BAD ABOUT INFLAMMATION

So just how does chronic inflammation lead to cancer development and promotion? The answer lies in the relatively new field of "Cell Signalling" which I'll briefly explain in a minute, but first the good news about inflammation is that it is not always a bad thing. In fact, our entire system of immune protection against invading pathogens such as viruses, bacteria, fungi and parasites, depend on immune cells generating inflammation by producing high levels of free radicals and immune chemicals called *cytokines* to burn up these nasty invaders.

Healing of injuries also depends on this immune system. When we bruise our finger, for example, the redness, swelling and pain associated with the resultant inflammation is the result of a complex biochemical cascade of events set in motion by the body's immune system in its attempt to repair the damaged tissue. These signalling molecules tell dormant stem cells to invade the injury, to proliferate and replace damaged cells and heal the injury. It's an amazing process that is usually short-lived and self-limiting.

However, when the inflammatory process continues for too long, or in an excessive or uncontrolled manner, it will become destructive to the DNA of stem cells resulting in gene mutations and chromosomal damage that transform them into cancer stem cells. These same pro-inflammatory signalling molecules that are used by the immune system to repair wounds also promote cancer growth and metastases. And, that's why any type of long standing inflammation is linked with a higher risk of developing cancer.

Fortunately the good news is that chronic inflammation is relatively easy to quench if you follow a few simple rules in relation to a healthy diet and lifestyle. In my book, *"Getting healthy naturally"*, I list the various dietary, lifestyle and systemic factors that cause chronic inflammation. Some we already know such as viral, bacterial and parasitic infections, as well as chemical irritants like tobacco smoke and non-digestible particles like asbestos.

## Other factors that cause ongoing inflammation include:

- Dietary factors, such as high sugar consumption, processed foods with their food additives and hydrogenated fats.
- Nutritional deficiencies (i.e. vitamins, minerals, amino acids, essential fatty acids).
- Environmental toxins, such as; heavy metals, industrial chemicals, pesticides, herbicides, chlorine and fluoridated water.
- Intestinal toxicity resulting from digestive dysfunction.
- Food sensitivity including food allergy and food intolerance.
- Lifestyle factors, for example, a sedentary life or the other extreme, excessive exercise, which generates high levels of free radicals.
- Long term stress and fixated negative emotions.
- Lack of quality sleep.
- Overweight and obesity.
- Immunosuppressant drugs.
- Radiation of all kinds such as nuclear, ionizing, ultraviolet light, or long term exposure to electro-magnetic fields.

## To Sum Up:

Our modern diet and toxic environment coupled with daily stresses and lack of exercise are some of the key areas we need to contend with in order to lower inflammation in our body tissues as quickly as possible. In the following chapters I will show you the many ways you can quench this insidious inflammation and in the process protect and enhance your immune system so it can effectively deal with any rogue cancer cells.

# THE EMOTIONAL CONNECTION TO CANCER

Dr Edward Bach (1886 – 1936) the English physician best known for developing a range of remedies called the Bach Flower Remedies believed that all diseases are in essence the result of conflict between the soul and mind of mankind, and will never be eradicated except by spiritual and mental effort.

In the early 1930's he wrote: "Behind all disease lie our fears, our anxieties, our greed and our likes and dislikes." [28]  He made this revolutionary statement upon personal observation of his many patients, whose physical ailments seemed to be predisposed by negative psychological or emotional states such as fear, anxiety, worries, jealousy, poor self image, anger and resentment. He believed that for true healing to occur, these negative emotional states must be resolved otherwise they will re-demonstrate their presence in another disease form at a later date.

It is generally accepted that cancer is usually the culmination of a number of factors, which also include things such as fear, insecurity, anxiety, frustration or anger that can also bring on cancer symptoms.

It is well known that different psychological states can trigger the release of certain glandular secretions in the body.  The mechanisms behind these secretions represent the connection between the mind and the body and these mechanisms have received intense scrutiny from medical researchers over the past thirty-plus years. This has led to a new field in medicine called psycho-neuroimmunology where studies have confirmed that the emotional and psychological state of a person influences a myriad of bodily processes for better or for worse.

Dr Douglas Brodie, MD (1925–2005) was an early pioneer in mind/body connection to cancer, and over the course of 50 years of treating many thousands of cancer patients, observed that there were certain personality traits and stressors that were consistently present in these patients. Here are the seven key traits that he discovered to be part of the cancer etiology: [29]

1. Being overly conscientious, dutiful, hard-working, caring and above average intelligence.

2. Taking on other peoples burdens and going that extra mile to one's own detriment (worries for others).

3. A people pleaser with a great need for approval.

4. Poor relationship with one or both parents, resulting in lack in intimacy with spouse.

5. Holding on to toxic emotions such as anger, resentment and hatred and not being able to express them.

6. An inability to handle life's stresses culminating with an especially traumatic event about two years before cancer is detected.

7. Inability to let go of emotional hurts usually arising in childhood, and oftentimes being unaware of their presence.

Dr Ryke Geerd Hamer (1935–2017), a renowned German physician and cancer surgeon claimed to discover proof of the mind/body connection to cancer through his first-hand experience. He was recovering from testicular cancer which he felt was somehow related to a traumatic event in his life. The event was the death of his son Dirk, who had been shot and subsequently died in his father's arms some time later. Soon after that event he developed testicular cancer which he identified as the result of a "Lost conflict". *(30)*

From this experience and as Chief Internist in a gynaecology-oncology clinic at Munich University, he was able to interview and examine the records of thousands of patients with reproductive organ cancers. He observed that they all had very similar traumatic events in their lives, a few years prior to the diagnosis of their cancer.

Dr. Hamer hypothesised that cancer originates from a shock or trauma that catches an individual completely by surprise. This traumatic event would initiate a sequence of events that simultaneously affect the psyche, the brain and corresponding body organs. His research led him to identify via CT scans, the presence of concentric rings in the emotional reflex centre of the brain as being evidence of the psycho-emotional trauma on the brain itself.

At the time of the traumatic experience, Dr. Hamer contends that the shock affects a specific area in the brain causing a lesion (concentric rings) to appear, which in turn sets off a sequence of events that weakens a particular organ leaving it susceptical to developing cancer. He proposed that the location of the newly formed lesion on the brain, which is seen through a CT scan, is like a map that can reveal the type of disease and its organ-location in the body.

In other words, he claimed that specific types of conflict (i.e. traumas, stresses, beliefs, etc.) can create specific kinds of disease states in the body including cancer. He also believed that the exact nature of the conflict predetermined which part of the brain and specifically which brain circuits would be affected.

He was able to confirm this hypothesis on the emotional level (by knowing the actual conflict), the physical level (the organ manifesting the corresponding disease) and on the brain level (confirmed by a CT scan).

In his own words Dr. Hamer stated: *"I searched for cancer in the cell and I have found it in the brain."*

---
## CHAPTER 2
---

# Contrasting Conventional Oncology with Naturopathic Oncology

*"Aggressive therapies are used when a Doctor is not skilled enough to make the most of gentle therapies"* – Dr. Isaac Elias

## RADIATION AND CHEMOTHERAPY'S DARK SECRETS

One of the most closely guarded secrets that oncologists and pharmaceutical companies keep is that most conventional cancer treatments actually cause cancer themselves and leave patients at risk of developing totally different secondary cancers. By damaging the DNA of normal cells, radiation and chemotherapy drugs heighten the risk that those cells will become cancerous at some point in the future.

It has been documented that anywhere from 5 to 17% of patients who undergo conventional treatments will develop a new cancer. For example, some breast cancer survivors will develop leukaemia.

Most cancer patients trust their oncologist out of either blind faith or fear of abandonment. Yet there is mounting evidence that the conventional treatments your doctor is recommending might actually make cancer grow faster and become incurable when used alone.

Cancer survival statistics are never based on a comparison of alternative against conventional treatments, but rather on the correlation between various conventional treatments, and protocols. By manipulating these statistics, oncologists and drug companies can give the impression that they are significantly extending

> The rationale for chemotherapy and radiation is that cancer is an enemy that must be killed or destroyed, even when the treatment causes the person great discomfort, perhaps even death. Chemotherapy drugs originated out of mustard gas, designed as a poison for use in warfare. No wonder chemotherapy is feared almost as much as cancer itself.

life for the cancer patient, when in fact it is all smoke and mirrors.

A group of researchers looked into the statistical benefits, if any, that chemotherapy has on increasing the likelihood of surviving cancer for more than five years. The researchers searched the literature for all the randomized clinical trials that reported a five-year survival benefit in adult cancers that could be attributable only to the chemotherapy they had been treated with. Here's what they found.[1]

*"The overall contribution of curative and adjuvant cytotoxic chemotherapy to five-year survival in adults was estimated to be 2.3% in Australia and 2.1% in the USA."* They go on. *"As the five-year relative survival rate for cancer in Australia is now over 60%, it's clear that cytotoxic chemotherapy only makes a minor contribution to cancer survival."* So what does that all mean?

What the researchers are telling us is that the data shows that 97% of the time that a patient with cancer lives past 5 years it is because of factors other than the chemotherapy they received. What could those other factors be? And why is the cancer industry only interested in chemotherapy instead of these other factors?

The other factors, as I've mentioned already include diet, lifestyle, detoxification, environment, supplementation etc. And the basic reason that they are not embraced by conventional oncology is that none of them are patentable. None of them are profitable.

Anytime a therapy that only has a 2.1-2.3% chance of having a long-term positive effect while at the same time being extremely toxic, I'm thinking that such a therapy needs some help. Sure, chemotherapy can be effective in the short haul. It might increase survival for another one to two years. But in order for a long-term survival, the other factors are needed.

So the lesson here is quite clear. Pay attention to other factors. If you have cancer, make sure you consult with an experienced Naturopath who can help you get on a detoxification program, an exercise program and the right diet and supplements.

## Why 75% of doctors would refuse chemotherapy on themselves

Polls and questionnaires show that three doctors out of four (75%) would refuse chemotherapy for themselves because of its ineffectiveness against cancer and its devastating effects on the body and the immune system.

> "The body is not crying for radiotherapy or chemotherapy. The body is crying to heal itself with nature." – Dr. Selvam Rengasamy

Polls were taken by accomplished scientists at the McGill Cancer Centre from 118 doctors who are all experts on cancer. They asked the doctors to imagine they had cancer and to choose from six different "experimental" therapies. These doctors not only denied chemo choices, but they said they wouldn't allow their family members to go through the process either! [2]

## This is what many other doctors and scientists have to say about chemotherapy:

*"The majority of the cancer patients in this country die because of chemotherapy, which does not cure breast, colon or lung cancer. This has been documented for over a decade and nevertheless doctors still utilize chemotherapy to fight these tumours."* (Allen Levin, MD, UCSF, "The Healing of Cancer", Marcus Books, 1990).

Dr. Hardin Jones, lecturer at the University of California, after having analyzed statistics on cancer survival for many decades, has come to this conclusion: *"when not treated, the patients do not get worse or they even get better."* The unsettling conclusions of Dr. Jones have never been refuted. (Walter Last, "The Ecologist", Vol. 28, no.2, March-April 1998)

*"Many oncologists recommend chemotherapy for almost any type of cancer, with a faith that is unshaken by almost constant failures."* (Albert Braverman, MD, "Medical Oncology in the 90s", Lancet, 1991, Vol. 337, p. 901)

*"Our most efficacious regimens are loaded with risks, side effects and practical problems; and after all the patients we have treated have paid the toll, only a minuscule percentage of them is paid off with an ephemeral period of tumoural regression and generally a partial one"* (Edward G. Griffin "World Without Cancer", American Media Publications, 1996)

*"After all, and for the overwhelming majority of the cases, there is no proof whatsoever that chemotherapy prolongs survival expectations. And this is the great lie about this therapy, that there is a correlation between the reduction of cancer and the extension of the life of the patient."* (Philip Day, "Cancer: Why we're still dying to know the truth", Credence Publications, 2000)

*"Most cancer patients in this country die of chemotherapy."* - Dr Allen Levin, "The Healing of Cancer", Marcus Books, 1990

*"A six or twelve-month course of chemotherapy not only is a very unpleasant experience but also has its own intrinsic mortality... Treatments now avert perhaps 2 or 3 percent of the 400,000 deaths from cancer that occur each year in the U.S."* - Prof John Cairns, Scientific American, Volume 253, No.5, 1985.

*"To sell chemotherapy as a 'therapy' is most likely the biggest deceit in the history of medicine. Whoever masterminded this chemo-torture deserves a monument in hell."* – Dr. Ryke Geerd Hamer, M.D.

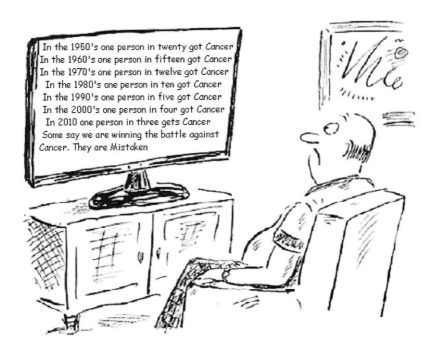

Everybody knows that chemotherapy drugs fill the body with horrific toxins, but because the medical regulatory body's outlaw doctors from suggesting or prescribing vitamin supplements, herbs and super-foods; this archaic chemical therapy is still recommended. The best way to beat cancer is to detoxify the body and build up the immune system, not break it down further by dosing one tumour with chemicals that pollute the entire body.

At best, chemotherapy should be considered an *"alternative"* treatment, but for the past 100 years allopathic medicine has warped the public perception of true (i.e. naturopathic) medicine.

So if you ever get a cancer diagnosis and your doctor tells you what to do, you may want to ask him/her if they would do the same thing for themselves and their family members.

Conventional treatments can actually make cancers more aggressive, more likely to spread, and more resistant to these conventional treatments.

Most chemotherapy agents do things such as:

- Stimulate inflammation mechanisms
- Increase free radical generation
- Promote angiogenesis
- Suppress anticancer immunity
- Promote cancer cell resistance to being killed

Radiation treatments also stimulate inflammation, increase free radical generation, and increase cancer cell resistance.

# NATUROPATHIC MEDICINE AS A VIABLE TREATMENT FOR CANCER

*"Most allopathic doctors think practitioners of alternative medicine are all quacks. They're not. Often they're sharp people who think differently about disease."* – Dr. Mehmet Oz

Most people are aware of the conventional methods of treating cancer, namely surgery, chemotherapy and radiation being the big three. In recent years, several other oncology therapies have made an appearance. Immunotherapy, Laser therapy, Photodynamic therapy and Stem Cell Transplants are all examples showing promising results. Yet, conventional oncology mostly adopts a reductionist approach to treatment, where one looks for a fundamental mechanism that causes or promotes cancer. For example, with breast cancer one tests to find out if it is hormone-dependent. If so, the treatment (after surgery) would focus on blocking those hormones with a pharmaceutical agent.

For some cancers this reductionist approach can be effective. For example, in the case of early stage melanoma (malignant skin cancer) if it is fully excised in time, the patient will most likely be cured. However, most cancers are quite complex and systemic in nature, meaning that if not treated in a holistic manner they will most likely recur with little chance of the allopathic approach being successful second time round.

The reason for this is that allopathic medicine doesn't address all the underlying causes contributing to the development of cancer. It is not enough to just target the tumourous lump without recognizing and dealing with the fact that the cancer is often a whole body problem that needs a multi-faceted treatment approach. Localized treatment may sometimes be needed but addressing the whole person (mind, body and spirit) would result in a higher likelihood of treating the root cause more effectively to fully eliminate cancer from the body.

This is an area where naturopathic medicine excels. Otherwise known as naturopathy it is a multi-disciplinary approach to healthcare that recognises and supports the body's innate power to heal itself. Naturopathy formulated what is now known as the five cornerstones of good health: sunshine, fresh air, exercise, sensible diet and a positive mental attitude. Drawing on ancient Greek philosophy, it set up as its basic concept the idea of the 'Vital Force'. To the Naturopath, the vital force pervades all of nature, keeping it in order and harmony. It is also present in the human body and shows as the body's innate power to heal itself.

Naturopaths see the symptoms of disease as the remedial effort of the body to throw off disease. They maintain it is an eliminative and cleansing process instituted by the body in an effort to rid itself of the accumulation of toxins. Properly managed, the disease process is also the road to cure.

## PRINCIPLES OF NATUROPATHIC MEDICINE

To give the body the best chance for self-healing, naturopaths operate within the guidelines of six time-tested principles:

1. **FIRST DO NO HARM:** By using only safe and effective medicinal substances and therapies that are not injurious to the patient, naturopaths are committed to the principle of causing no harm.

2. **NATURE'S HEALING POWER:** The human body is governed by, and when injured, restored by the action of an invisible agent called the Vital Force and the role of the naturopath is to aid that force in restoring its equilibrium with the aid of natural, non-toxic substances, as well as the removal of obstacles to healing and recovery.

3. **IDENTIFY AND TREAT THE CAUSE:** Naturopaths do not seek to suppress symptoms, but to discover and remove the root cause of disease, whether it be physical, psychological or spiritual.

4. **TREAT THE WHOLE PERSON:** Naturopaths operate within a holistic philosophical framework, treating the whole person rather than just a disease or one part of the body. They have a deep understanding that illness occurs on many levels and so, take into account individual physical, mental, emotional, social, environmental and other factors. Since total health also includes spiritual health, naturopaths encourage individuals to pursue their personal spiritual development.

5. **THE PHYSICIAN IS A TEACHER:** One of the aspects of the therapeutic approach of a naturopath is to guide and educate the patient in developing a healthier lifestyle.

6. **PREVENTION IS THE BEST MEDICINE:** Remember the old saying *"an ounce of prevention is worth a pound of cure."* Naturopaths don't wait for disease to progress before they institute appropriate preventative measures in partnership with their clients to prevent illness.

Naturopathy as a healing modality has much to offer in this present day and age of "techno medicine". Naturopathic medicine can be applied in any healthcare situation, but its strongest area is in the treatment of chronic and degenerative diseases including cancer. You see, the more one studies the causes of the common diseases of our age, the more apparent it becomes that the answer doesn't lie in treatment methods that rely purely on suppression or the learn-to-live-with-it variety, particularly in the chronic diseases of the elderly. The answer lies in finding the underlying causes of ones health problems, and then dealing effectively with them in order to return the patient to full health. This is very important for cancer in both terms of treatment and prevention.

## 'How do I know if Naturopathic Medicine is Right for Me?'

This is a question that many of our patients ask when they are considering the best ways to reach their health goals and overcome chronic health concerns. This bullet point list will clearly help you determine if we can help you:

- I am interested in getting to the root cause of my health concerns and don't want to just put a 'band-aid' on them.

- I want to experience relief and healing without side effects.

- I want my entire quality of health and life to improve - not to just feel a little bit better in one specific area of my body.

- I want a healthcare team that truly cares about me and is committed to helping me experience lasting healing and well-being.

- I don't want to be rushed through the healthcare process.

- I want healthcare providers that will really listen to me.

- I struggle with chronic health issues that have not responded very well to conventional medical approaches.

- I am not sick or unwell, but I just know that my health could be a whole lot better.

- I feel like I don't know how to manage stress very well.

- I'm ready to make lasting lifestyle changes and will do whatever it takes to finally feel fully alive.

- I know that investing in my health is one of the most important priorities in life.

If any or all of these statements describe you, then there's an excellent chance that we can help! Keep reading so you too can enjoy the amazing and profound benefits that naturopathic care has to offer.

# THE COMPLETE CANCER TREATMENT PLAN

Cancer is now the number one cause of death in western countries. It is a vicious disease that invades the body with abnormal tissue growth and eventually strangles its victims with malnutrition (cachexia), infections, or multiple organ failure. When it comes to treating cancer we need a "comprehensive" approach, which incorporates both natural medicine as well as conventional approaches in order to overcome this formidable enemy. We should not discard any cancer therapy, no matter how strange to prevailing medical theories it appears, unless that therapy does not produce results.

Conventional treatments like radiation and chemotherapy are good at killing cancer cells and shrinking tumours, but they also kill healthy cells. In the process, they wipe out one of our greatest allies in the cancer battle - your immune system. Once your body defences are damaged, then you are in a worse position than before because in the end, your immune system is going to be the only thing that saves you. Protecting your defence mechanisms is probably the most critical reason you need to incorporate natural remedies like vitamins and herbal medicines into your treatment protocol.

There are no "magic bullets" against cancer so it's generally best to hedge your bets both ways. You can do both conventional and holistic therapies in conjunction. Obviously, all cases are different, so I can only outline my general principles and approach when treating cancer clients.

When treating cancer clients I take a four-pronged approach:

## 1. **Reduce Tumour burden**:

We need to remove or debulk the tumour if possible using surgery, restrained chemo and radiation, which can remove as much as 10 trillion cancer cells and give the cancer patient's system a fighting chance.

- Surgery has its place, especially when the tumour has been encapsulated and can be removed without rupturing the collagen envelope.

- Chemotherapy can be useful, especially for certain types of cancer and when administered in small doses to a well-nourished patient. Modern chemical treatments for tumours are becoming more specifically targeted and not as dangerous as old time chemotherapy.
- Radiation therapy has its place, especially as the highly-targeted brachytherapy or intensity-modulated radiation therapy (IMRT).

## 2. **Protect your Body from the Effects of Chemotherapy and Radiation**:

Many oncologists tell you not to take any antioxidants (e.g. vitamins A, C and E) or herbal supplements while you're undergoing chemo or radiation. This baffles me, because published studies show patients who combine nutritional therapies with chemo or radiation do better

> One of the greatest virtues of naturopathic medicine is its ability to greatly diminish, if not eliminate, these side effects and thereby improve the chances for a full and enduring recovery.

than patients taking no supplements while undergoing these treatments. For example, a study review in Cancer Treatment Reviews looked at 845 articles published on taking antioxidant supplements such as vitamins A, C and E, glutathione, melatonin, ellagic acid and N-Acetyl - cysteine while undergoing chemotherapy.

Researchers found that in many cases, patients taking antioxidants had increased survival times, increased tumour responses, or both. They also had reduced toxic side effects from the chemo when compared to patients not taking supplements. [3] That's why I use plenty of supplements and herbs in my cancer protocols.

3. **Build Your Overall Health and Immune System:**
   I tell my cancer clients that if they want to beat cancer, they have to become "the healthiest person on the block". Unfortunately, by the time someone has cancer, their overall health is seriously compromised. Therefore, we need to apply nutrition and other naturopathic fields to bolster immune function in the cancer patient to reverse the underlying cause of the disease, and to nourish the patient's recuperative powers.

4. **Address the Root Cause of Cancer:**
   This is the part that most oncologists never treat. It's not enough to kill the cancer and strengthen your immune system; you also have to address what caused the cancer in the first place. If you don't address the underlying causes, the cancer will just come back.

Cancer rarely has just one cause. It is often caused by a combination of factors, including genetics, carcinogen exposure, toxicity buildup, pathogens, dietary deficiencies, hormonal imbalances, decreased energy production in your cells, and psychological factors.

Dangerous toxins like heavy metals, pesticides, pollutants and other chemicals are one cause. They're in the air we breathe, the water we drink, and the food we eat. These toxins build up in our tissues and organs and slowly poison our body. So one thing you must do is start a serious detoxification program. This could involve dietary change, fasting, using saunas and taking herbal tonics. When you take all four steps, you have a much greater chance of beating cancer for good.

# THE GOOD NEWS

The best treatment for cancer would be to find a way to make cancer cells revert back to being normal cells - a process called *"redifferentiation"*. That would make the cancer disappear without having to kill cancer cells. It would be completely painless and nonmutilating to the body and might only involve swallowing some special pills.

Believe it or not there are some natural compounds that have differentiation properties. For example, the vitamin A component, All-trans Retinoic acid (ATRA) converts malignant leukaemia cells back to normal white blood cells. (4) This same vitamin compound also seems to cause malignant melanoma cells to differentiate into normal pigment cells.(5) In another study they found that an extract of licorice also strongly stimulated melanoma cells to differentiate. Apigenin, a flavonoid abundant in many fruit and vegetables such as oranges, grapefruit, onions and parsley also promotes differentiation of malignant skin cells.(6)

Vitamin D3 has also been shown to strongly stimulate differentiation in acute myeloid leukaemia cells. Unfortunately, high-dose vitamin D3 can cause blood calcium levels to rise dramatically, which can lead to medical problems. However, one particular study found that adding rosemary extract (which is high in carnosic acid) could greatly enhance the cancer cell differentiation effect of vitamin D3, even when D3 is used in doses low enough not to cause calcium elevation.(7)

Silibinin, an extract from milk thistle, has been shown to keep prostate cancer cells from becoming undifferentiated cancer cells.(8) Flavonoids from grape extracts were shown to stimulate differentiation of colon cancer cells.(9) N-butyrate, a short chain fatty acid produced by bacterial fermentation in the gut was shown to be the most powerful stimulator of differentiation especially for colon cancer cells. (10)

Curcumin, a bright yellow extract found in the spice turmeric was shown to promote differentiation of glioma (brain) cells.(6) And a final example, hesperidin, a flavonoid compound found abundantly in citrus fruits has been shown to induce differentiation in thyroid cancer cells.(11) All of these plant extracts are available in concentrated form without prescription.

If these natural substances have such powerful anti-cancer effects, why aren't doctors using them to treat cancer? There are several reasons I suspect:

- The most obvious reason is that the benefits of these natural remedies lie buried beneath a growing mountain of drug company profits. The pharmaceutical industry is making billions of dollars off traditional treatments and they do not want to lose these profits. So this long-standing "conflict of interest" has kept a great number of alternative treatments from wide-spread use. What if the cure for cancer can't be made in a lab!!

- Another reason is because allopathic medicine has been monopolized by the pharmaceutical industry and as such, doctors receive no real training in nutrition or herbalism and so have no understanding or clinical experience with these therapies. Medical doctors' main focus is by and large, in the use of pharmaceuticals and surgery.

- Another reason doctors and oncologists don't know about these natural compounds is because they do not generally read scientific journals where these natural compounds are most often discussed. They prefer clinical trials which mostly carry articles about allopathic treatments and are heavily sponsored by pharmaceutical companies. In addition, most medical conferences are sponsored by pharmaceutical companies, so the programs presented are biased towards allopathic treatments.

## DEALING WITH CONVENTIONAL DOCTORS

Should you choose to follow an alternative treatment approach to conquer your cancer, you'll be going against the grain of modern conventional oncology. One difficulty that can arise as a result of this is the difficulty involved with declining the modern treatment your oncologist thinks you should get. Most people with cancer are first diagnosed by a conventional doctor. If you are one of these people, you may have seen an oncologist who is very committed to the mainstream "accepted" approaches. It is no easy task to turn down a medical specialist's recommendation – especially when you may be told that, in doing so, you will be killing yourself. One thing to remember in this situation is that, specialist or not, *your doctor works for you.* You are paying your doctor for their expertise and professional service. It is important to listen to and consider any recommendations for treatment your doctor gives you. But when it comes to the final decision you make, that is up to you.

If you choose to follow an alternative approach, you may be in a situation where you still want to see your conventional doctor at certain intervals for diagnostic monitoring. Even people using alternative methods will still want to have blood tests, CT scans, or other tests done regularly to ascertain their progress. Or there may be side complications of your cancer that you will want to go to a conventional doctor for help with at times.

I recommend being as open as possible with your conventional doctor. It is best to be honest and to give your doctor the opportunity of deciding to follow your progress while you use an alternative approach. You may be surprised to find that your doctor is more open-minded than you expected. If, however, your doctor takes a stance against alternative approaches and will not prescribe diagnostic tests to you unless you undergo conventional treatments, then you have the option of finding another doctor or oncologist who will. I recommend that you make an effort to find a doctor with whom you can work openly. In doing so, you are also emotionally standing up for yourself and your right to choose your own treatment.

## The Takeaway

We know toxic treatments such as chemotherapy and radiation aren't the answer. Doctors even know better than anyone how devastating chemo can be. According to one report, when a leading doctor at the famous Sloan-Kettering Cancer Center found out he had advanced-stage cancer he told his colleagues, do anything you want but no chemotherapy!

You need to know that you have options that exist beyond

mainstream medicine and big pharma. Don't use the one-size-fits-all model that currently exists. You can select a treatment that works for you. Trying non-conventional therapies has brought success to many cancer patients. This includes those who received conventional medicine's advice to *"go home and plan your funeral!"*

If you are diagnosed with cancer it's crucial to have an oncologist who is willing to listen to you and work with you. Make it a team effort. It's not a dictatorship. And you always have options.

It's time to ask for more than the standard protocol. You deserve treatment that doesn't make you sick. We've all seen people on chemo. Some of us have experienced it. It's very ugly. The gold standard should be a treatment that boosts the body, not a cell-destroying poison. One size does not fit all. So, in the following chapters I'll show you how to stack the deck in your favour.

---
## CHAPTER 3
---

# Let Food be Your Medicine

*"Let food be your medicine, the body will heal itself."*
Hippocrates – The Father of Medicine

*He that takes medicine and neglects diet and nutrition wastes the skill of the physician.* – Chinese Proverb

**N**o disease is more vicious than cancer. It kills many hundreds of thousands of people across the globe every year. And the deaths are often long, drawn-out and painful. When it comes to treating cancer no one approach is always successful. Conventional treatments like chemotherapy may be good at killing cancer tumours but they also kill healthy cells, and the treatment in itself is also carcinogenic. In addition, the process also wipes out one of your greatest allies in the cancer battle - your immune system.

The bottom line is that if you want to stand a chance of beating cancer you can't just rely on the allopathic approach of slash, burn and poison. You have to do a comprehensive approach that takes the best of both worlds. And that's where nutrition plays a major part in any anti-cancer treatment plan. For instance with nutrition we know through pharmacokinetics (the study of the action of a substance within the body) that vitamins A, C, and E are regulators of cell differentiation, cell membrane integrity and DNA synthesis. Studies show that these nutrients are toxic to cancer cells. They stimulate the immune system, up-regulate DNA repair, inhibit angiogenesis (the formation of blood vessels in tumours) and augment apoptosis (programmed cell death).

## THERAPEUTIC NUTRITION CAN:

### 1. Prevent and/or Reverse Malnutrition

Most cancer patients don't die from the cancer itself. They die from being worn out and wasted. This condition is called **CACHEXIA**. Cachexia is the gradual wasting away of a cancer patient's body, often to just skin and bones. That's because the cancer is stealing the nutrients (mostly glucose) from the rest of the body. Patients literally starve to death.

Fortunately, there's a way to block this wasting away and that's to make sure your body is getting enough super-nutrition, high in all the vitamins, minerals and phytonutrients essential to 'health'. Many oncologists to this day are hesitant to recommend to their patients higher levels of nutrients, fearing they could also feed the cancer and make it grow faster. However, to dispel this myth, a few intrepid researchers tried feeding terminal cancer patients high nutrient diets. They discovered two things; the patients lived longer; and their tumours did not grow any faster. Since then, a great number of similar studies have confirmed these initial findings.

### 2. Protect your body from the toxic effects of chemotherapy and radiation

Many oncologists advise you not to take any antioxidants or supplements while you're doing chemotherapy and radiation. They say this in the mistaken belief that antioxidants will neutralize or reduce the effectiveness of chemo and radiation. Yet there are many published studies that show patients who combine nutritional supplements with conventional treatment do better than patients doing conventional alone. Properly nourished patients experience less nausea, vomiting, weakness, immune suppression, hair loss and weight loss. Conventional allopathic treatments also seem to work much better alongside nutritional treatments.

Essentially, the proper selection of nutrients taken before and during chemotherapy and radiation can help make the allopathic therapy more of a selective toxin against the cancer. In one study reported in the Journal of Clinical Oncology, cancer patients were either given vitamin E at 300mg per day or a placebo while undergoing cisplatin (chemo drug) therapy. Only 31% of the vitamin E group developed neurotoxicity, while 86% of the placebo group developed neurotoxicity.*(1)*

Another 2007 study in Cancer Treatment Reviews looked at 845 articles of randomized controlled studies evaluating the effects of concurrent use of antioxidants and chemotherapy. The antioxidants used in these studies included vitamins A, C and E, glutathione, melatonin, ellagic acid and n-acetyl-cysteine. These antioxidants did not negatively interfere with the chemotherapy; on the contrary, they were associated with increased survival time, increased tumour responses and less toxicity as compared to those patients on chemotherapy alone.*(2)*

## 3. Boost your Immune System

If your immune system is weak, it can play a major role in cancer activation. Poor nutrition and nutrient destroying cooking methods only serve to weaken the immune system even further. A healthy diet, on the other hand, supports the immune system. This support comes in the form of nutrients. If the diet isn't supplying those nutrients, the body struggles to work properly. At least 40% of annual cancer deaths can be partially attributed to diet.*(3)* If you want to beat cancer, you have to become optimally nourished in order to have an immune system strong enough to fight off all pathogens as well as seek out and destroy cancer cells.

## 4. Cancer's Sweet Tooth

Most people don't realize this and the medical establishment rarely addresses it - but sugar feeds cancer cells! It's simple; sugar (glucose) is the preferred fuel source for cancer cells. In addition, the over consumption of sugar increases insulin levels and promotes inflammation, both of which promote cancer growth.

Cancer cells need glucose to fuel their growth, and they take it up at a rapid rate. This is because they have many more receptor sites on their cell walls for glucose uptake than normal cells have. They also metabolize glucose differently than normal cells as I explained in Chapter One. This altered glucose metabolism is very energy inefficient meaning they need lots of glucose for fuel.

Doesn't it stand to reason therefore, that if sugar feeds cancer and we were to remove this food source, most cancer cells would die! Why then is this knowledge being so dramatically overlooked by the medical establishment?

Instead of them encouraging their cancer patients to eat a diet of sugary foods in a misguided attempt to prevent weight loss, they should be severely restricting simple carbohydrates and all sugars and instead, encouraging their patients to eat a low-protein, high-fat diet known as a ketogenic diet. I'll go into greater detail on the ketogenic diet in other chapters.

## 5. Inhibit Cancer Growth

Many nutritional compounds and phytochemicals found in foods and herbs have the capacity to inhibit cancer cell growth. Some of these nutrients can even help convert cancer cells back into normal cells, a process called re-differentiation. Some of the most powerful nutrients in this category are the carotenoids such as alpha-carotene, beta-carotene and lycopene. Foods rich in these carotenoids include red, orange and yellow fruits and vegetables such as tomatoes, carrots, apricots, red and yellow peppers.

In order for tumours to grow and spread, cancer cells have developed the ability to secrete certain enzymes that allow them to spread. Several nutrients have the capacity to block the action of these enzymes, thereby preventing the growth and spread of cancerous tumours. Foods that contain these nutrients in therapeutic amounts include citrus fruits like oranges, lemons and grapefruits.

Tumours also need a blood supply to survive and grow. The process of growing new blood vessels from existing blood vessels is called ANGIOGENESIS. Cancer researchers have developed drugs that can block angiogenesis; however, they always come with unwanted side effects. Inflammation within the body promotes angiogenesis so a diet based primarily on anti-inflammatory foods will reduce inflammation and help inhibit angiogenesis. Omega-3 fish oils, especially the DHA component have been shown to reduce angiogenesis.

The plant flavonoids luteolin and apigenin, which are found in high concentrations in globe artichokes, celery, parsley, onions and leeks also inhibits angiogenesis, as well as promoting re-differentiation of cancer cells back to normal cells. Other plant compounds that exhibit anti-angiogenic properties and re-differentiation traits include curcumin, quercetin and hesperidin and can all be bought as supplements.

## BEATING CANCER WITH NUTRITION

Cancer is an extremely lucrative business for large pharmaceutical companies who produce drugs to treat the disease so they're not always forthcoming with suggestions on nutrition, the right food choices and the use of special nutraceutical supplements in their fight against cancer. The good news however, is that nutrition can make a huge difference in the outcome of

In most medical schools, students receive only a few hours of instruction on nutrition. As a result, most new doctors have little knowledge of the power of nutrition against disease and are discouraged from thinking along these lines and consequently do not incorporate nutrition in their practices.

your cancer treatment. Many people are blown away when they see the results a few simple dietary changes can make, not just in their fight against cancer, but in their general health and wellbeing. Nutrition, on its own is not always sufficient but it is essential, meaning no-one should use diet as a sole therapy against cancer. However, let me emphazise: diet along with nutritional supplementation is an essential component of everyones comprehensive cancer regime.

Nutrient deficiencies, which are prevalent today, can contribute to an overall weakening of the body and its immune defences, making a person more vulnerable to cancer onset. Today, medical and research journals that deal with cancer are filled with studies confirming what holistic physicians have long known: diet and nutrition are both at the core of cancer etiology and its successful treatment. A well nourished cancer patient can better manage the disease and its varied therapies. Most cancer sufferers will get a dramatic improvement in quality and quantity of life and much better chances for a complete remission.

A healthy human body is self-regulating and self repairing. The fact is that if you are healthy, you are constantly beating cancer. According to America's National Institutes of Health, the average adult gets cancer about six times in their lifetime, but are able to defeat it because they have innate mechanisms within their body that help to defeat and eliminate cancer; and nutrition is an important part of nourishing those mechanisms. With optimal nutrition you can re-regulate your body and positively change its host defence mechanisms to find and destroy the cancer.


## SO MANY DIETS!

We've got a lot of confusion today, about what we should eat for health. There are people who say we should eat only vegetarian or vegan, others profess the merits of the macrobiotic diet or paleo-diet. Still, others suggest a diet based on low carbohydrates and high in fat, (The Atkins diet and ketogenic diet). And to add more confusion there are those who swear by a low-fat, high-fibre diet (Pritikin diet). There are literally dozens of variations to those diets, so how is one to make sense of it all.

Well, if we look at the medical research on nutrition and cancer, and understand cancer cell metabolism then it becomes quite clear that there are clear guidelines on what foods to eat and which ones to avoid. The simple truth is there are dangerous foods, which promote cancer development and spread, and there is a clear biochemical basis for this. What we know without a shadow of doubt is that we need to eliminate as much as possible sugar in all its forms. For over 90 years we've known that cancer is an 'obligate glucose metaboliser' (Sugar feeder). (4) Indeed, it has been argued that most cancer cells would die if starved of sugar.

About 90 years ago, a Nobel Prize - winning scientist named Otto Warburg discovered exactly what feeds cancer. (5) As you may already know, the cells in your body use one of two types of fuel. They burn either glucose (sugar) or Ketones (fat). But Warburg showed that cancer cells live almost entirely on glucose. Their defective metabolism means they can't convert fat into energy.

Warburg proved this by showing that cancer cells create a tremendous amount of a by-product called lactic acid as a result of fermentation. Scientists have known for a long time that lactic acid isn't produced when a cell burns fat; it's only produced when a cell inefficiently burns glucose as all cancer cells do. Because of their defective cellular machinary, cancer cells also depend on glucose to fix any damage caused by free radical production and lipid perioxidation products. These unstable molecules are formed in the body as a consequence of cellular metabolism. As the cancer cell's mitochondria (power generators) aren't working properly, they must rely even more on the uptake of glucose to counteract this oxidative damage. All of which means that cancer cells rely a lot on glucose for their survival.

So, the best way to starve cancer out of your body is to avoid all foods that significantly increase the amount of sugar in your bloodstream. That means staying away from sugar, starchy foods like potatoes, beans, cereals, breads, pasta and other refined carbohydrates. Just remember sugar comes in many different guises such as dextrose, maltodextrin, agave, fructose and corn syrup, so you need to become sugar-wise and learn to read labels. Better still, aim to eat only real foods and preferably organic.

Avoid all processed foods; I'm talking about isolated, purified, extracted etc - there are so many ways to create what I call fake or "franken foods". A simple rule to follow, if it's God-made, eat it (example butter) and if it's man-made, dustbin it (eg margarine). So when you start to exclusively eat real foods and only real foods such as organically grown fruits and vegetables, nuts and seeds, etc, you'll start a healthy foundation and your body will begin to do exactly what you want it to do.

Eating organically grown foods is extremely important as many studies have shown that these foods are free of carcinogenic contaminants, unlike conventionally grown foods. They are also richer in the essential nutrients necessary for cancer prevention, including beta-carotene, vitamin E and selenium. In addition, fresh organic vegetables, especially green-leaf vegetables and their juices, as well as beetroot and wheatgrass juice have been shown to be able to improve the oxygen metabolism of cancer cells helping to make them less malignant and possibly even revert them to normal cells.

Additionally, it is essential you avoid highly processed foods as they usually contain hydrogenated fats as well as various chemical additives, which are potentially carcinogenic. Cancer-causing foods include those that contain pesticides, herbicides, fungicides, chemical additives, added sugar or artificial sweeteners; also processed meats, burnt (barbecue) foods, fried foods and all junk foods. Some examples include deli meats, sausages, chips, hot dogs, charred, smoked or cured meats, ice cream, white rice and refined grains, sugary and artificially sweetened drinks, and processed vegetable oils, which are high in hydrogenated fats.

## A WORD ON FATS

Fats have gotten a lot of negative press over the years. Cardiologists are always warning people to avoid foods containing cholesterol, as well as foods high in saturated fats and every other source of fat except, ironically, the one group most associated with poor health - Omega 6 fats (more on that later).

Most people, including doctors, think of "fats" as either saturated fats or unsaturated fats, which is further broken down to omega-3 fats (found in fish oils) or omega-6 fats (found in vegetable oils). They forget about other types of fats such as:

- monounsaturated fats (high in olive oil and avocado oil)
- medium chain oils (found in coconut oil)
- short chain fats (fermented by gut bacteria and also made in the liver: ketones)

Lipid (fat) chemistry is, in fact, very complex, and lipids have a number of powerful biochemical and physiological effects. They can act like powerful drugs - either beneficial or harmful.

## Fats: The Good and the Bad

Fats have been shown to play a major role in the etiology of cancer. Some fats help prevent it while others promote its growth and ability to spread. I call these "good fats" and "bad fats".

We've all heard about omega-3 and omega-6 fatty acids and how essential they are to health. They have important roles in many body systems. They are converted into hormone-like substances called eicosanoids. Eicosanoids derived from omega-6 fats tend to promote inflammation, while those derived from omega-3 fats are anti-inflammatory in nature. The roughly opposing actions of omega-6 and Omega-3 fatty acids mean that it is more important to balance their intake.

Unfortunately, with today's food choices, our intake of these fats is quite imbalanced with the average person consuming a much higher ratio of omega-6 to Omega-3 fatty acids. Studies show that we on average have 15 to 20 times more omega-6 than omega 3 in us, while the recommended ratio for omega-6 to omega-3 is set at 2:1.[6] This imbalance of omega 6/3 together with getting too little omega-3 in our diet is connected to different unfavorable health conditions such as an increased inflammation level and a reduced immune function.*(7)*

Excess consumption of omega-6 fats have been shown to contribute to many chronic and life-threatening conditions including cancer, heart disease, Alzheimer's disease, and autoimmune diseases.*(8)* A number of experiments have revealed that omega-6 fatty acids work as an activator for cancer, making it grow and spread more easily. They achieve this through a number of mechanisms, one of which is by increasing the COX-2 enzyme.

Research also clearly shows that high levels of omega-6 fats can drive the beneficial omega-3 fats out of cells and tissues. So, the only healthy solution is to significantly reduce our intake of omega-6 fats and increase our intake of the omega-3 fats and their derivatives EPA and DHA.

Omega 6 fats are found in abundance in polyunsaturated vegetable oils such as:

- Sunflower
- Safflower
- Canola
- Soya bean
- Palm
- Peanut
- Corn
- Rapeseed

Foods that contain these oils are often rancid or oxidized, which makes them even more harmful to the cancer patient. Most processed foods contain one or more of these oils. Also, keep in mind that virtually all processed foods such as bread, cereals, desserts, chips, taco shells and many salad dressings are cooked in large vats of omega 6 oils. You should only ever cook with monounsaturated oils such as extra virgin olive oil, coconut oil or avocado oil.

# HYDROGENATION

The process called hydrogenation is where hydrogen atoms are forced into polyunsaturated oils under high pressure and temperature in order to turn the oils into fatty solids. These fatty solids are then made into margarines, shortening, and used widely in the confectionery industry. The oils get changed at the molecular level during the hydrogenation process resulting in the creation of trans-fatty acids. These trans-fatty acids do not occur in nature and so cannot be properly metabolised and used within the body.

However, these man-made toxins end up being incorporated into cell membranes where they can cause havoc with cell metabolism. They block the proper utilization of essential fatty acids, thereby inducing cellular dysfunction and promote ongoing inflammation. *(9)* Not only has the consumption of hydrogenated (trans) fat been implicated in the development and spread of cancer, but also, a host of other chronic life-threatening conditions such as heart disease, diabetes, obesity neurological diseases and autoimmune diseases.*(10)*

The newer margarines, while lower in hydrogenated fats, are still made from cheaply produced rancid vegetable oils such as rapeseed, soy, corn or canola and contain many additives. Your best defence is to avoid all hydrogenated products like the Plague.

# HEALTHY FATS

The good fats include Omega-3 fatty acids found abundantly in oily fish, and other oils that are converted into EPA (eicosapentaenoic acid) and DHA (docosahexaenoic acid) such as alpha-linolenic acid from flaxseed. The Omega-3 fatty acids come from algae, which explains how fish obtain them. This is also why farm-raised fish are devoid of omega-3 fats, which are composed of two valuable nutrients EPA and DHA.

Of the two, DHA has the more powerful anti-cancer effect and it is especially good at preventing cancer of the colon, prostate and breasts.*(11)* Pure DHA is derived from algae and an adult's dose is 500 mg a day. DHA has been shown to inhibit cancer using a number of mechanisms, but primarily by reducing inflammation.

When taking fish oils, make certain that the label says it contains both EPA and DHA. And remember that these oils should be kept refrigerated at all times. Good sources of omega-3 fats are found in cold water fish including wild Alaskan sockeye salmon, mackerel, trout, herring, sardines, anchovies, crab and scallops.

Because seafood often contains significant levels of mercury and other pollutants such as PCB's, dioxins and pesticides I've deliberately listed only those that are naturally low in these toxins and heavy metals.

Plant sources of omega-3 fats include flaxseeds and acai berries, which are composed of alpha-linolenic acid that our bodies can convert into EPA and DHA. A word of caution: do not use flaxseed oil as it tends to be oxidized and gone rancid; and therefore is dangerous. Instead put your whole organic flaxseed and acai berries in smoothies.

---

**The skinny on fats**
Keep this list handy - it will help you identify good fats and bad.

**Healthy fats**
- Extra virgin olive oil
- Omega-3 fats (fish oil, DHA, EPA and flax seeds)
- EPA (eicosapentaenoic acid)
- DHA (docosahexaenoic acid)
- Gamma-linolenic acid (GLA) - borage oil
- Conjugated linolenic acid (CLA)
- Extra-virgin coconut oil
- Avocado oil

**Unhealthy fats**
- Omega-6 oils (corn, safflower, sunflower, peanut, canola, and soybean)
- Trans-fatty acids (partially hydrogenated oils).

---

---
**CHAPTER 4**
---

# The Ketogenic Diet Starves Cancer

*"Sugar is the most hazardous foodstuff in your diet"* – Linus
Pauling, PhD, twice Nobel laureate

I hold the view, along with numerous health experts that the vast
majority of cancer cases are preventable and also curable. To achieve
success, the key here is to view cancer as a metabolic dysfunction,
which needs to be properly addressed in order to gain control over this
devastating disease. Simply put the right choice of foods along with
other strategies will help suppress cancer growth while simultaneously
pushing it into remission.

As I explained elsewhere, cancer cells are unlike normal cells in
many ways, but one of their traits that is unique relates to insulin
receptors. They have 10 times more insulin receptors on their
membrane surface. This enables cancer cells to gorge themselves with
glucose coming from the bloodstream at a very high rate. If you
continue to consume foods like carbohydrates and sugar as your
dominant food source, cancer cells will continue to thrive and spread.
It is a known fact that the lowest survival rate in cancer patients is
among those who have high blood glucose levels. What most people

don't know is that cancer cells are mainly fueled by glucose: in this regard, the ketogenic diet is logically the best dietary approach. By depriving cancer cells of their primary source of fuel, as well as protein restriction (cancer cells also feed off glutamine, an amino acid) cancer cells will literally starve to death.

## WHAT IS THE KETOGENIC DIET?

Many of you may have heard about the ketogenic diet and how it can potentially starve cancer into oblivion. There have been many experiments in which animals with cancer showed a striking decrease in cancer growth when they were put on a ketogenic diet. *(1)*

### What is Ketosis

Ketosis is a metabolic state in which the body uses dietary fat and body fat stores as its primary energy source. Normally the body operates in a state called "glycolysis" where it derives its energy from glucose (sugars and carbohydrates). When in a state of ketosis, the liver breaks down fat and short-chained fatty acids called ketones, which can be used by body cells for energy production. The adoption of a ketogenic diet forces the body to adapt to using ketones for energy through dietary deprivation of the foods that provide glucose, namely sugar and simple carbohydrates.

Simply put, a ketogenic diet is one that all but completely eliminates carbohydrates, restricts protein, while at the same time increasing dietary fat. This type of diet switches your metabolism from glucose-burning to fat-burning. This is called ketosis.

You can starve cancer cells by sticking to a ketogenic diet consisting of an abundance of healthy fats, such as avocados, organic eggs, cold water oily fish, raw nuts and seeds, butter, coconut and olive oils etc. Percentage-wise the diet should be 75% fats, 20% protein, and no more than 5% carbohydrates. One of the fastest ways to prevent or knock your metabolism out of nutritional ketosis is by consuming sugar or high-glycaemic carbohydrates; which of course is not what we want to do!

Much research regarding the ketogenic diet in relation to fighting cancer has grown over the years, and the evidence suggests that the reason ketogenic diets have such a dramatic effect on cancer growth, is that by limiting carbohydrates and excess proteins, you can actually STARVE the cancer cells.

As you probably know by now all your body cells are fuelled by glucose. This includes cancer cells. However, cancer cells have one built-in fatal flaw; they do not have the metabolic flexibility to adapt from using glucose for fuel to using ketone bodies which come from the breakdown of fats - hence the name "ketogenic".

As glucose is the main fuel used by cancers for growth, the diet works by lowering blood sugar and insulin, while at the same time stimulating the liver to break down dietary fats into special high energy molecules called ketones. Healthy cells can use either glucose or ketones as their energy source, but cancer cells only use glucose in this case.

Another reason the ketogenic diet works so effectively against cancer is because unlike normal cells, cancer cells require both glucose and insulin to grow. Dietary glucose reduction not only reduces insulin levels but also reduces circulating levels of the growth hormone IGF-1, which is necessary for driving cancer cell metabolism and growth. [1] IGF-1 (insulin growth factor) is a potent hormone that acts on the pituitary gland to stimulate metabolic and endocrine effects including cell growth and cell division. Elevated levels of IGF-1 are associated with breast and other cancers. [2]

As I mentioned earlier, cancer patients with high blood glucose levels experience rapid tumour growth and metastasis. High glucose levels also promote angiogenesis (new blood vessel growth within a tumour) which is essential for tumour growth and invasion. Drug companies are always searching for drugs that inhibit angiogenesis because such inhibition would powerfully inhibit cancer growth. Yet, ironically, many oncologists tell their patients to eat lots of sugary carbohydrates to prevent weight loss during therapy.

The aim of the ketogenic diet is to shift you from a glucose-burning metabolism to a fat-burning metabolism. Now get this: The ketones that the diet produces have a direct toxic effect on cancer cells. *(3)* Also, we know that cancer cells have defective mitochondria (powerhouse of the cell that converts glucose or ketone bodies to energy, ie; ATP) and according to ketogenic experts energy metabolism leads to the production of harmful reactive oxygen species (ROS) molecules. Glucose is essential to destroying these (ROS molecules), so if one is already on a glucose-restrictive (ketogenic) diet, these ROS molecules will kill the cancer cells.

Ketones also have a powerful anti-inflammatory effect on the body. Inflammation is a major underlying cause of cancer initiation and spread, making it grow like wildfire.*(4)* By drastically reducing the intake of sugar and refined carbohydrates not only is inflammation reduced, this type of diet also improves macrophage immune function.*(5)* Macrophages are the main immune cells directing the body's attack against cancers.

Ketones also inhibit harmful enzymes that promote cancer cell growth and cancer invasion.

One such enzyme is called histone deacetylases (HDAC). Research has demonstrated that ketones that inhibit HDAC reduce cancer cell growth, activate tumour suppressor genes, and promote normal cell division. *(6)*

---

**KETOSIS AND KETOACIDOSIS: THE DIFFERENCE**

Ketosis and ketoacidosis, though similar in name, are extremely different metabolic states.

**Ketosis**, as defined in this chapter, is a state in which the body "flips" from utilizing carbohydrate for energy to using fat. This happens through dietary deprivation of carbohydrate, which creates a regulated and controlled amount of ketones in the body.

**Ketoacidosis**, on the other hand, is a dangerous metabolic state brought on by a lack of insulin in the body and the presence of massive quantities of ketones. This state is usually seen in type 1 diabetes, and it should be monitored closely by anyone suffering from the disease.

As you can see, there are a number of benefits from following a ketogenic diet:

- Starvation of cancer cells

- Toxic effect on cancer cells

- Reduction of inflammation

- Inhibition of angiogenesis

- Suppression of harmful enzymes

- Improvement in immune function

It's of interest to note that the most common link found in healthy centenarians is a low-calorie, low-protein high-fat diet combined with regular exercise. This diet and exercise lifestyle confers a moderate elevation of ketones throughout their life.

Sounds good so far; but here's the problem. Although the ketogenic diet does indeed slow down the growth of cancers, it doesn't completely starve them. That's because in addition to sugar and insulin, cancer cells can also use the amino acid glutamine as a fuel for growth. Also, diets that are high in protein are also capable of feeding cancer because high-protein drives the MTOR pathway, which causes cancer cell proliferation. So that's the reason a low to moderate protein intake is recommended on the ketogenic diet in order to weaken cancer cells.

What if it were possible to block cancer cells from using glutamine as a fuel? Then maybe, we could completely starve cancer while on a ketogenic diet. Fortunately, cancer researchers have discovered certain natural compounds that stop cancer cells from being able to use glutamine.

Cancer cells take up glutamine primarily through a transporter protein called ASCT2. ASCT2 levels are highest in lung, breast and colon tissue, which explains why cancers in these regions are the most aggressive, fastest growing and fastest spreading cancers. A recently published study in the journal of Precision Oncology has discovered three natural compounds that starve cancer cells via inhibition of glutamine uptake by cancer cells. [7] Scientists from the University of Texas did experiments on mice injecting them with cancer cells, allowing a tumour to form. They then fed the mice a diet that contained various combinations of cucumin, ursolic acid and resveratrol. They discovered that all three compounds had strong cancer-killing properties. But they were even more powerful when used in combination.

The study explained the mechanisms by which these three natural compounds working synergistically on a cellular level can block glutamine uptake by cancer cells. Without this food source cancer cells will die. So, if you were to combine these compounds with a ketogenic diet, such a combination will deprive cancer cells of not only glutamine, but also glucose and insulin. This is literally everything they need to survive and grow. And, while all this is happening, the normal healthy cells will be unaffected.

Here is a list of the foods highest in these three cancer-starving compounds:

**Curcumin**: Turmeric powder, the bright yellow spice commonly used in Indian curry. Curcumin is better absorbed if you combine it with a little bit of black pepper, and also good oils, making it more absorbable.

**Ursolic Acid**: Apples (especially the skin), cranberries, prunes, olive oil, basil, lavender, oregano, peppermint, sage and thyme.

**Resveratrol**: Red grapes, blueberries, dark chocolate, red grape juice and red wine.

You should incorporate as many of these foods into your diet and also take a daily supplement containing these three ingredients.

This type of diet, whereby you restrict all but non-starchy vegetable carbohydrates and replace them with low to moderate amounts (10 to 20%) of high quality protein and high amounts (60 to 80%) of beneficial fats is what I recommend for everyone, whether they have cancer or not. It's a diet that will help optimise your weight and all chronic degenerative disease, as eating this way will help you convert from a glucose-burning mode to a fat-burning mode.

# ADVICE ON IMPLEMENTING A KETOGENIC DIET

To implement a ketogenic diet, the first step is to take a look at what you're eating and start to eliminate anything that's unhealthy. That means staying away from sugars, processed and packaged foods, starches, sweet drinks, chocolate, ice cream and cheap polyunsaturated oils. The key culprits in processed foods include polyunsaturated fats, hydrogenated (trans) fats and added sugar in all its forms especially glucose and fructose, as well as refined carbohydrates. Artifical ingredients added into the mix can also promote inflammation.

Furthermore, stop drinking cow's milk because it contains the sugar galactose. Drinking just one glass can use up your entire allowance for the day. I also recommend avoiding all dairy products as the protein casein in dairy can also trigger inflammation in individuals who are sensitive to it. And, as I have already explained, inflammation is not only a major cause of cancer development, it also drives the cancer, making it grow faster and spread. Dairy products also have very high levels of glutamate, which is made from glutamine - a tumour growth promoter.

# KETOGENIC ESSENTIALS

The ketogenic diet consists of a meal centred around healthy fats. While calories from non-fibre carbohydrates should be virtually eliminated, calories from protein just need to be reduced to get a more ideal ratio of fat to protein. This diet does not mean totally eliminating carbohydrates. You need to have plenty of fresh organic fibre-filled vegetables (complex carbs). That means you can eat several hundred grams of vegetables per day as the fibres will be converted to short-chain fatty acids by friendly bacteria in the gut, which in turn drives ketosis.

Protein intake should be restricted to 1.2 grams per kilogram of body mass. Remember, eating excessive protein can trigger cancer growth by stimulating the MTOR pathway, which accelerates cancer growth.

As regards dietary fats, you need to increase them by 70-80% and only consume healthy fats. These include:

- Avocados
- Organic eggs
- Omega-3 rich fish including wild caught alaskan salmon, mackerel, herring, sardines, scallops, anchovies, rainbow trout
- Nuts such as brazil, pine nuts, hazelnuts, macadamia, almonds and pecans.
- Seeds such as flax, hemp, chia, acai, sesame and pumpkin
- Grass-fed organic meats and wild game
- Extra-virgin olive oil, coconut oil, avocado oil and macadamia oil
- Kerrygold butter

When implementing the ketogenic diet, I recommend you get two servings of healthy fats with every meal. For example you could add a tablespoon of olive oil to your salad, which includes a medium avocado.

Protein sources in a ketogenic diet generally come from:

- Fish
- Meats
- Poultry
- wild game
- nuts
- legumes

Also, when implementing your ketogenic meal plan, it's imperative to stick to green leafy vegetables because they are rich in fibre as well as health promoting nutrients and phytochemicals, many of which have anti-cancer properties. Your best choices include:

- Cabbage, especially purple
- Broccoli

- Cauliflower
- Brussels sprouts
- Spinach
- Kale
- Leeks
- Yellow and red onions
- Garlic
- Beetroot and beet leaves
- Green and red peppers
- Celery
- Asparagus
- Zucchini
- Parsley
- Carrots

While fruits are a healthy food group the majority of them should be avoided while on a ketogenic diet because of their high amounts of sugar. However, certain berries are beneficial and safe to eat in moderate quantities including blueberries, blackberries, strawberries, raspberries, grapes, cranberries and pomegranates, because they are rich in antioxidants and many other cancer-fighting nutrients that can support your health.

Again, I will reiterate how important it is to refrain from eating any simple carbohydrate foods and sugar in all its forms. Remember even honey is 50% glucose and 50% fructose! The ketogenic diet involves the use of non-starchy carbohydrates only.

As for beverages the most important is WATER (purified only). Green tea should be drunk daily as it is rich in EGCG, a potent anticancer flavonoid. Coconut water is very hydrating and some of the nut milks will have beneficial nutrients as well.

## SUPPLEMENTS THAT ENHANCE KETOSIS

When you embark upon the ketogenic diet it is recommended to supplement it with high quality vitamins and minerals, probiotics, and omega-3 fatty acids. 150mg of resveratrol a day has been shown to have the same benefits as weekly fasting (more about fasting later). By taking probiotics you enhance your production of Butyrate in your colon. Butyrate is a short-chain fatty acid that is a potent inhibitor of HDAC. Research shows that chemicals and compounds that inhibit HDAC, reduce cancer cell growth, activate tumour suppressor genes and promote normal cell division. *(6)*

Omega-3 supplementation with this diet also amplifies its anti-cancer effects. Adding medium-chain triglycerides (MCT) to meals is one way of increasing the amount of healthy fat in this diet. Coconut oil is high in MCT, or you can buy pure MCT oil in your local health food store. A teaspoon twice-daily should be sufficient.

## THE IMPORTANCE OF INTERMITTENT FASTING AS AN ADJUNCT TO THE KETOGENIC DIET

*"I keep my health by dieting. People gorge themselves with rich foods, use up their time, ruin their digestion and poison themselves... If the doctors would prescribe dieting instead of drugs, the ailments of normal man would disappear. Half the people are food drunk all the time. That is the secret of my health."* - Thomas Edison

Besides increasing healthy fats, limiting protein and restricting carbohydrates, you can also strengthen your ketone engine with intermittent fasting. Fasting increases ketone production, putting further pressure on starving cancer cells.

Intermittent fasting involves an individual scheduling their meals in such a way that they get a period of fasting each day. This involves eating all their meals within a six to eight hour period, which means they're fasting for 16-18 hours each day. This regular intermittent fasting lifestyle upregulates the enzymes that are designed to burn fat as a fuel, and downregulates the glucose enzymes.

You can implement intermittent fasting by starting off by not eating for 3 hours before you go to bed and then gradually extend that time to five or even six hours. So, by not eating between 6p.m. and 10a.m. the following morning you give yourself a window of 16 hours without food.

When I first started intermittent fasting, I decided to skip breakfast. But I soon realised that it's not a good idea to eat late in the evening (especially a heavy meal), because that's when your body is preparing for rest, repair and regeneration. Eating a meal in the evening results in a higher insulin response as opposed to eating the same meal in the middle of the day. Insulin response is what drives a lot of weight gain in addition to generating excessive amounts of damaging reactive oxygen species (ROS).

On a side-note; when talking about food intake in relation to its metabolism, I like to describe it as a "build-up phase" and a "cleaning phase". The build-up phase is the time between your first meal of the day, and your last meal of the day, and your cleaning phase is the time between your last meal of the day and your first meal the next day. In our society today, with the amount of environmental toxins that we are exposed to, including what's in our food, it's imperative that we move towards doing a 2:1 ratio of cleansing to building. That means having your last meal around 6pm and breakfast the next morning at around 10am, which gives you a 16 hour fast. 'As you move towards that ideal ratio and you continue to practice the principles of a ketogenic diet, you will see better and better health results. You will literally look and feel younger five years from now, than you do now by applying intermittent fasting.

One of the best things I tell all my cancer clients, whether they elect to do conventional cancer treatment such as chemotherapy and radiation, or combine them with natural therapies, is to do intermittent fasting combined with a Ketogenic diet. From my perspective, I believe it's nothing short of medical malpractice and negligence to fail to integrate this type of dietary strategy into a patient's cancer treatment plan. A Ketogenic diet along with intermittent fasting can be easily integrated into whatever cancer treatment plan you decide to follow. And more over, research has shown that fasting this way helps chemotherapy deliver better results, with less side-effect and less need for the heavy doses usually given. Indeed, I strongly recommend this dietary strategy for everyone, whether they have cancer or not, as a burst of new research support fasting, along with calorie reduction as a life span extender.

## FASTING TO BEAT CANCER

*"I fast for greater physical and mental efficiency."* - **Plato**

*"A little starvation can really do more for the average sick man than can the best medicines and the best doctors."* - **Mark Twain**

*"The best of all medicines is resting and fasting."* - **Benjamin Franklin**

*"Fasting is the greatest remedy - the physician within."* - **Philippus Paracelsus**

Fasting is one of the oldest dietary interventions in the world for the treatment of illness, and now modern science confirms it's beneficial influence on a person's health. Over history, wise men, prophets and other key leaders fasted. Fasting is prescribed in the Bible and is considered a path to physical and spiritual purity. Anyone who is a Christian knows that Jesus fasted for 40 days in preparation for his ministry. Hippocrates was quoted as asserting *"Instead of using medicine, rather fast a day."*

Before I get into greater detail and the benefits of fasting let's take an historical look at this strategy's most basic form taken to the extreme....

**FORTY TWO DAYS WITHOUT FOOD: How One Doctor's Desire to Die Revealed Fastings Supreme Benefits for Life!**

Henry Tanner, M.D., a respected, middle-aged physician from Duluth, Minnesota had reached the point in his life where he no longer wanted to live. Spending his waking hours in pain, he had suffered from rheumatism, asthma and disrupted sleep for years.

All the doctors he consulted considered his case "hopeless". Back in those days in medical school, Tanner learned that the human body could survive without food for only 10 days. With that fact in mind, he created his "death plan". He would simply stop eating and at the end of 10 days his misery would be over.

But, to his amazement, his intentions didn't go as planned... By the fifth day of his fast, Tanner was sleeping more peacefully. And instead of dying by day 10, he felt as well as he did in his youthful days. Continuing to fast until day 42 and by now under a fellow physician's supervision - Tanner surprised himself and proved his naysayers wrong. His symptoms of rheumatism, asthma and chronic pain were gone. Dr. Tanner went on to live a full life until he died at the age of 87. [8]


## THE BREUSS CANCER CURE

One of the most well-known healers in the last century to employ fasting as a treatment for cancer was a man called Rudolf Breuss. He is reported to have cured over 50,000 cancer sufferers over his long career as a healer. [9] Breuss maintained that cancer feeds off protein to grow and spread. (N.B. This is not fully accurate in the light of what we know today about cancer).

He therefore deducted that if one fasted for an ideal period of 42 days, taking only a blend of vegetable juices, along with herbal teas to detoxify, cleanse and eliminate toxins, the cancer would starve, be absorbed and subsequently pass out of the body and be eliminated.

A man ahead of his time, this was radical thinking that flew in the face of the accepted medical wisdom of the day but it is now used all over the world and known as the Breuss Total Cancer Treatment.

# THE BREUSS JUICE

Raw vegetable juices have long been used in natural medicine as part of the healing system for many chronic conditions. Raw juices contain antioxidants, anticancer phytochemicals, and living enzymes that science has identified as an imperative part of everyone's diet if they wish to stay strong and healthy. It is against this backdrop that Bruess developed his cancer treatment protocol, utilising the healing properties of vegetable juices and herbal teas that have been associated with the cure of many types of cancer.

The Breuss Juice consisted of a specific mixture of organically grown beetroot, carrot, celery, potato and radish juices. This mixture, provided in liquid form all the vitamins and minerals required by the body during the 42 day fast, whilst the body's own innate healing resources are used in dealing with the cancerous tumours. Multiple testimonials attested to the success of this treatment in curing cancer.

It's interesting when I first tell people about fasting and its health benefits, they're super sceptical. They think it's a terrible idea. Apart from claiming they could never do it, they also believe that they'd be super hungry all the time as well as having no energy or strength to carry out their daily activities or work. But the opposite is true, as I can attest to from the numerous fasts I completed ranging from 10 to 20 days. What happens during fasting is that after a few days of fasting, your basal metabolic rate increases when your body switches from glucose-burning to fat-burning. Once it starts burning body fat its like, hey! There's plenty of this stuff, Lets burn our 2,000 calorie daily needs....

**Benefits of Fasting**

- Increased energy
- Upregulated immunity
- Enhanced liver function
- Reduced allergy symptoms
- Increased metabolism
- Weight loss
- Improved digestive function
- Reduced aches and pains
- Reduced inflammation
- Improved sleep
- Reduced food cravings
- Heightened mental clarity
- Feeling of calmness and mental stability

This is why fasting tends to increase energy as opposed to leaving you feeling drained. If you're overweight and lethargic, fasting helps unlock all that energy already lodged in your body that you previously had no access to. Fasting forces your body to start accessing those stores of energy, and once that happens, your body suddenly has a near unlimited supply of energy. When you start to use up some of your fat stores you won't feel hungry because you're in essence eating your own fat. That's one thing my clients are always surprised about. When they come back they say: "Hey, I'm not actually that hungry." That's no surprise because their body is feeding off their own stored fat and so it doesn't need to eat.

## SEVERAL MECHANISMS INVOLVED IN FASTING

Many factors are at work during fasting, including enhanced autophagy (breakdown of old damaged cells), less aggressive hormone production, glucose deprivation and low insulin levels. Sirtuin stimulatim is increased. Sirtuins are protective hormones known to be produced under conditions of food deprivation. One of the most notable benefits of fasting is its profound anti-inflammatory effect. Fasting increases production of anti-inflammatory cytokines while at the same time suppressing the production of pro-inflammatory cytokines. Pro-inflammatory cytokines are associated with insulin resistance (a precursor to diabetes), obesity and a shorter lifespan, whereas anti-inflammatory cytokines are associated with improved insulin sensitivity, improved fat burning, increased muscle regeneration and a longer life span.

**Autophagy**: Autophagy is a natural occurring process in the body involving the breakdown of old damaged or abnormally developing cells so that their components can be recycled for normal healthy processes and to make new healthy vibrant cells.

Autophagy is derived from the Greek words meaning "'self-eating".

It's like taking out the trash... This vital cleanout process detoxifies your cells and recycles the parts that are no longer needed. Autophagy also destroys foreign invaders such as viruses, bacteria and other pathogens.

We know that cancer formation and chronic degenerative diseases are marked by inefficient autophagy processes. When our body is able to efficiently breakdown old damaged cells and use the components to make new healthy cells, we are going to protect genomic integrity (DNA). By creating a stronger healthier cell, when that cell divides and continues to replicate, it's going to have healthy offspring, rather than an older cell that's damaged being allowed to continue to replicate and possibly turn cancerous.

There may be multiple ways to boost autophagy but none compare to fasting. When you allow your body to go without food, your cells trigger your innate autophagy switch.

## Fasting improves insulin sensitivity:

People even when they're not hungry, are forcing themselves to eat something. This excess food consumption desensitizes the cells to insulin in an effort to avoid the stress of a heavy calorie intake. This results in elevated blood insulin levels that lead to increased fat storage; all of which causes increased oxidative damage and resultant inflammatory conditions within the body (cancer thrives on inflammation). Increased insulin also enhances cellular division which is a risk factor for cancer formation. When insulin is high, our body's store fat and autophagy (breakdown of old damaged cells) processes decrease.

## Fasting Increases Human Growth Hormone (HGH) Levels

HGH is the quintessential anti-aging hormone. HGH and insulin are opposites in function. HGH is focused on tissue repair, efficient fuel usage and anti-inflammatory immune activity. Researchers at the Intermountain Medical Centre Heart Institute in Salt Lake City, Utah found that men who had fasted for 24 hours had a 2,000% increase in circulating HGH, while women who were tested had a 1,300% increase in HGH. The researchers also found the fasting subjects had significantly reduced their triglycrids (blood fats), boosted their good cholesterol (HDL's) and stabilized their blood sugar. *(10)*

## Fasting helps Chemotherapy

Studies on people and animals have shown that short periods of fasting helps chemotherapy deliver better results and with less side effects. Dr. Valter Longo and colleagues at the University of Southern California have shown that a 48 hour fast protects normal cells in mice with cancer tumours undergoing chemotherapy, but not the cancer cells.

The researchers also published a study on ten cancer patients who voluntarily fasted for a short-term (1-6 days) before and after chemotherapy. The patient's reported far fewer side effects from chemotherapy such as less weakness, nausea and less fatigue. The same team produced further research showing that fasting makes cancer cells more sensitive to chemotherapy. Fasting, they claimed stops cancer cells producing protective proteins, thereby increasing cancer's vulnerability to chemo while healthy cells on the other hand made more protective proteins. As a result, the healthy cells stop replicating and are therefore less vulnerable to attack by the chemotherapy, resulting in lower side effects.

But the team identified another factor working against cancer cells, namely that fasting deprives a cancer cell of glucose. Dr. Longo describes these as two stressors acting simultaneously. These USC scientists therefore suggest that fasting in combination with chemotherapy is feasible, safe and has the potential to ameliorate side effects caused by chemotherapies.(11)

## Contraindications to Fasting

While the majority of people would likely benefit from fasting, there are a few absolute contraindications. If any of the following apply to you, you should not do extended fasting:

- Underweight defined as having a body mass index (BMI) of 18.5

or less

- Malnourished (in which case you need to eat healthier more calorie dense nutritious food)

- Pregnant and breastfeeding women. The Mother needs a steady supply of macro and micro nutrients in order to assure the baby's healthy growth and development, so fasting is deemed too risky for the baby

- Children generally should not fast as they need a continual supply of nutrients for healthy growth. If a child needs to lose weight, a far safer and more appropriate approach is to eliminate sugars and simple carbohydrates from their diets.

---
**CHAPTER 5**
---

# Foods that fight Cancer

*If you want to reverse cancer without the person getting sicker, you need to give the body substances that selectively kill the cancer while strongly supporting the body's nutritional and immunological health* – Robert C. Atkins, M.D.

**W**hile doing research for this book on the health benefits of different foods, I ran across an absolutely jaw-dropping study that was done all the way back in 2008 and published in 2009, a study which in the website 'Chris Beats Cancer' *(1)* reports a 'cure' for many kinds of cancer has already seemingly been found.

From Chris's website: 'Chris Beats Cancer'a study was published in Food Chemistry, January 2009 called, "The antiproliferative and antioxidant activities of common vegetables: A Comparative study"*(2)*.

Researchers studied the inhibitory (cancer stopping) effects of 34 vegetable extracts on 8 different tumour cell lines. They basically just ran vegetables through a juicer and then dripped extracted juice on different cancer cells to see what would happen. Here are the top 10 anti-cancer vegetables from the study...

The no.1 most powerful anti-cancer food was garlic. Garlic stopped cancer growth COMPLETELY against these tumour cell lines: breast cancer, brain cancer, lung cancer, pancreatic cancer, prostate cancer, childhood brain cancer and stomach cancer. Rounding out the top 10 were: Leeks, yellow and green onions, broccoli, brussels sprouts, cauliflower, kale, red and curly cabbage, spinach and beetroot.

As his story pointed out, there are literally thousands of published peer-reviewed studies demonstrating that the 100,000+ phytonutrients in plants have the ability to prevent and reverse cancer. But because the pharmaceutical industry can't figure out how to extract these compounds, synthesise them, and patent them for profit, they are ignored.

And as Chris also points out, while it's important to keep in mind that this was only a laboratory study showing what various vegetable extracts did to cancer cells when applied directly upon them, the study did not take into account the vitamins, minerals and phytonutrients that indirectly support your body's ability to repair, regenerate, detoxify and heal, nor did it take into account an individual's daily routines or lifestyle, *"having said all that, it makes sense to focus on eating tons of the veggies that were actually killing cancer in the lab."*

And Chris Wark would know as he was diagnosed with stage III colon cancer in 2003. From his website: *"I was diagnosed with stage III colon cancer in 2003. After surgery I opted-out of chemo and used nutrient and natural therapies to heal. Today I'm healthy, strong and cancer-free! Also this study confirms why what I did in 2004 worked. I ate copious amounts of these cancer-fighting vegetables everyday in my giant Cancer-Fighting salad, (3) specifically spinach, kale, broccoli, cauliflower, onions, red cabbage, and garlic powder. I had no idea about leeks or else they would have been in there too."*

His story continues to this day and with a very happy ending, one that 'Big Pharma' surely doesn't want us to know about:

*"Garlic is an anti-cancer vegetable. And according to Dr. Richard Schulze's recommendation, I ate several cloves of garlic per day. If garlic kills cancer, then I wanted to saturate my body with garlic. So I would just crush up cloves and swallow them with a mouthful of water. I also*

*took kyolic garlic extract. And yes, I reeked, but I lived to tell the tale!"*

Critical to any plan to combat active cancers and prevent their recurrence is to change one's diet from the modern western diet high in omega-6 fats, sugars, processed food, and red meats, to one high in nutrient rich vegetables, fruits and good fats from fish, nuts and seeds. You should aim to eat at least 10 servings of nutrient-dense vegetables and fruits each day to attain the maximum therapeutic nutritional effect.

Of the best kept secrets hidden from the public is that Health and Cancer research institutes around the world have been conducting studies with vegetable and fruit extracts for years, discovering their remarkable cancer-fighting effects. Plants contain thousands of phytochemicals, the naturally occurring plant chemicals that fight cancer and protect you from many other kinds of disease. These chemicals provide plants with colour, odour and flavour. When we eat them, research shows they can influence the chemical processes inside our bodies in helpful ways.

One class of phytochemicals, the flavonoids, have remarkable powers that have been confirmed by a number of researchers and documented in most major oncology journals. These compounds not only treat disease, including cancer but can even prevent them from occurring in the first place. They can also enhance the ability of most chemotherapy drugs and radiation to kill cancer cells, while at the same time protect normal cells from their harmful effects. Unfortunately most oncologists reading these journals tend to skip over these studies, preferring to focus on traditional chemotherapy agents and newer protocols.

**In a nutshell, laboratory studies have shown that phytochemicals have the potential to:**

- Stimulate the immune system
- Block substances we eat, drink and breathe from becoming carcinogenic
- Reduce the kind of inflammation that makes cancer growth more likely

- Prevent DNA damage and help with DNA repair
- Reduce the kind of oxidative damage to cells that can spark cancer
- Slow the growth rate of cancer cells
- Trigger damaged cells to commit suicide before they can reporduce
- Help to regulate hormones (4)

The following chart from the American Institute for Cancer Research lists some of the phytochemicals attracting serious scientific attention, identifies food sources and outlines potential benefits.

## Phytochemicals

| Phytochemical(s) | Plant Source | Possible Benefits |
|---|---|---|
| Carotenoids (such as beta-carotene, lycopene, lutein, zeaxanthin) | Red, orange and green fruits and vegetables including broccoli, carrots, cooked tomatoes, leafy greens, sweet potatoes, winter squash, apricots, cantaloupe, oranges and watermelon | May inhibit cancer cell growth, work as antioxidants and improve immune response |
| Flavonoids (such as anthocyanins and quercetin) | Apples, citrus fruits, onions, soybeans and soy products (Tofu, soy milk, edamame, etc.), coffee and tea | May inhibit inflammation and tumour growth; may aid immunity and boost production of detoxifying enzymes in the body |
| Indoles and Glusocinolates (sulforaphane) | Cruciferous vegetables (Broccoli, cabbage, collard greens, kale, cauliflower and brussels sprouts) | May induce detoxification of carcinogens, limit production of cancer-related hormones, block carcinogens and prevent tumour growth |
| Inositol (Phytic acid) | Bran from corn, oats, rice, rye and wheat, nuts, soybeans, and soy products (tofu, soy milk, edamame, etc) | May retard cell growth and work as antioxidant |

| Isoflavones (daidzein and genistein) | Soybeans, and soy products (tofu, soy milk, edamame, etc) | May inhibit tumour growth, limit production of cancer-related hormones and generally work as antioxidant |
|---|---|---|
| Isothiocyanates | Cruciferous vegetables (Broccoli, cabbage, collard greens, kale, cauliflower and brussels sprouts) | May induce detoxification of carcinogens, block tumour growth and work as antioxidants |
| Polyphenols (such as ellagic acid and resveratrol) | Green tea, grapes, wine, berries, citrus fruits, apples, whole grains and peanuts | May prevent cancer formation, prevent inflammation and work as antioxidants |
| Terpenes (such as perillyl alcohol, limonene, carnosol) | Cherries, citrus fruit peel, rosemary | May protect cells from becoming cancerous, slow cancer cell growth, strengthen immune function, limit production of cancer-related hormones, fight viruses, work as antioxidants |

# BEST CANCER-FIGHTING PLANTS

As with most things in life, quality trumps quantity when it comes to choosing the best fruits and vegetables to help you beat cancer. While fruits can have important cancer-destroying nutrients I don't recommend you eat a lot of them. That's because most are high in sugar, which can promote cancer growth. Certain vegetables contain extremely high levels of cancer-inhibiting compounds while others have very few. For the purpose of this book we'll only be focusing on some of the very best cancer-fighting and immune boosting plants.

Following is a list and brief description of plants that each play a role in disabling one or more steps in the multi-step cancer process.

# DARK GREEN LEAFY VEGETABLES

Leafy greens are the cornerstone of any healthy diet since they're exceptionally rich in vitamins, minerals, antioxidants, enzymes and many phytochemicals. Many of these nutrients, especially the antioxidants are known to combat cancer including vitamin C and beta-carotene (a precurser of vitamin A).

A diet rich in greens will help alkalize your body. A slightly alkaline metabolism and body is preferable as it improves performance of your immune system, and research shows that cancer thrives best in an acidic environment. Some of the best leafy greens include spinach, kale, nettles, rocket leaves, watercrest, parsley, wheatgrass and barley grass.

## CRUCIFEROUS VEGETABLES

Cruciferous vegetables such as broccoli, cauliflower, brussel sprouts, asparagus and cabbage, especially the purple variety are among the most powerful cancer-fighting foods to be found. They are high in fibre vitamins, minerals and important antioxidants such as the carotenoids and sulforaphane compounds. Many are also rich in glutathione, known as the body's "master antioxidant", since it has high free-radical scavenging abilities. Nearly all members of the cruciferous vegetables are nutrient-dense sources of a family of phytochemicals called isothiocyanates, which help breakdown potential carcinogens. Isothiocyanates, which are made from gluosinolates have been reported to help detoxify your body at the cellular level.

In addition, cruciferous vegetables also contain indoles and especially indole-3 - carbinol which, along with its metabolite Di-indole methane (DIM) modifies and diminishes aggressive oestrogen action. Research shows that these indoles inhibit cancer growth by converting the strongest oestrogen, oestradiol into the weaker form oestriol. This change from strong to weak oestrogen prevents cancer cells from growing, and is especially useful for the treatment of oestrogen driven cancers. (5) Make sure to include plenty of these vegetables in your daily diet.

## BEETROOT AND BEET GREENS

There are some amazing health benefits packed into this vibrant vegetable. Besides being loaded with immune boosting vitamin C, fibre and essential minerals like potassium, iron, sulfur, manganese, and magnesium, beets are also high in other health-promoting compounds like antioxidants, caroteroids, nitrates and a compound called betanin, which gives beets their deep crimson colour, and has been shown to reduce tumours in both animals and humans. *(6)*

In the 1950's Dr. Alexander Ferenczi, a Hungarian Oncologist, began prescribing cancer patients a regime of raw and juiced beets in their diets. Patients ate up to 1kg of beetroot a day. According to reports these patients who were in the final stages of cancer all showed remarkable improvement in their conditions with tumours shrinking and disappearing fully. *(7)*

Beets aid health in many other ways too. They lower blood pressure via their naturally occurring nitrates; they increase levels of specific enzymes in the liver involved in detoxification and have been traditionally valued for their ability to detox and purify your blood and liver. They also alkalize the body and promote better digestive health.

## EAT THE BEET LEAVES TOO

If you throw away the green leafy tops on your beetroot, you're doing yourself a disservice as these are among the healthiest part of the plant. Besides containing important nutrients like fibre, protein, phosphorus, zinc, B-vitamins, magnesium, potassium, copper and manganese, beet greens also contain a good amount of vitamins A and C, the carotenoids lutein and zeaxanthin, as well as calcium and iron. All in all, beet greens actually have a higher nutritional value overall than the beetroot itself.

Beet greens can be added raw to salads, juiced along with the raw beetroot or, sauteed lightly along with other greens like spinach. I like to marinate them in olive oil with a squeeze of lemon juice and some culinary herbs.

## RED ONIONS

When it comes to cancer-fighting foods you have to know your onions, red onions in fact. They are the most effective in the onion family because they have two chemicals that kill cancer cells. They have high amounts of quercetin, a powerful flavonoid, and anthocyanin, the pigment that gives the onion it's red colour.

The high levels of quercetin are so effective at scavenging free radicals (unstable molecules) that it possesses the ability to prevent tumour cell growth. In addition, it is believed that the anthocyanin compounds can supercharge the quercetin and magnify it's scavenging powers. Anthocyanins also suppress a cancer cell's ability to grow and spread by inhibiting angiogenesis. By inhibiting angiogenesis, cancer cells cannot form tumours or spread to new areas of the body.

The high sulfur-containing amino acids of red onions also supports the body's natural ability to detox and reduce inflammation. Allicin is another anti-oxidant compound abundantly concentrated in red onions. Allicin is effective at destroying pathogens that weaken the immune response and support cancer development.

Overall, red onions promote an unfavourable environment for cancer cells to survive. They activate many pathways that disrupt cancer cell growth and encourage cancer cells to commit suicide.

To get the highest amount of nutrients from red onions, avoid over peeling the onion as the skin contains the majority of the anthocyanin content. The allicin compound is released only when the onion is chopped, so only chop up the onion a few minutes before adding it to salads and other recipes. Heat degrades many of the antioxidants in red onions so it is advisable to eat them raw as often as possible to optimize the beneficial nutrients you are consuming. Also, when cooking red onions, cook at a low temperature to limit nutrient loss.

## GARLIC

Like red onions garlic is a rich source of the potent anticancer bioflavonoid quercetin. Garlic also contains large quantities of the antiviral, antibiotic and antifungal compound allicin. This makes it especially useful in the treatment of cancer if the patients also have concurrent candida infections as a consequence of taking chemo drugs and antibiotics. Allicin has been shown to activate enzymes in the body that weaken and kill cancer cells without harming normal cells. Studies show that those who eat garlic regularly have much lower rates of breast, stomach and colon cancer. (8) Diallyl sulfide, compound in garlic oil has also been shown to destroy carocinogens in the liver.

Garlic is not only a cancer killer but as Sarah Landers had reported within this June of 2016 story over at Natural News, (9) garlic's healing properties are so intense that it is 100 times more effective than antibiotic treatments.

As this natural news story also points out, garlic is also anti-viral, anti-bacterial, anti-parasitic and anti-fungal and as of yet, various bacteria's that have grown resistant to antibiotics have not grown resistant to garlic.

From this Natural News Story: Garlic has been used for thousands of years all over the world, and modern science is now backing up its medicinal properties. A recent study by researchers at Washington University has found that garlic can be up to 100 times as effective at treating bacterial infections as most mainstream antibiotics. Garlic is not just antibacterial, but it is also packed full of antioxidants that work to improve your overall health. It is high in sulphur, which can help to detoxify your system and remove unwanted toxins as well as removing other substances that make your body more vulnerable to infection.

In closing, as of the moment of my assessing this information (August 2020), there have been 6,545 peer-reviewed studies that have evaluated garlic's ability to prevent and improve a wide spectrum of diseases including cancer, and do you know what all this research revealed? I'll close here with this excerpt from this January of 2017 story by Dr. Axe: (10)

Eating garlic regularly is not only good for us; it has been linked to reducing or even helping to prevent four of the major causes of death worldwide, including heart disease, stroke, cancer and infections. The National Cancer institute does not recommend any dietary supplement for cancer prevention, but it does recognise garlic as one of several vegetables with potential anti-cancer properties. As you are about to see, raw garlic benefits are plentiful. It can be used as an effective form of plant-based medicine in many ways, including the following:

1. Garlic for Heart Disease
2. Garlic for Cancer
3. Garlic for High Blood Pressure
4. Garlic for Colds and Infections
5. Garlic for Male and Female Hair loss (Alopecia)
6. Garlic for Alzheimer's disease and Dementia
7. Garlic for Diabetes

For maximum benefit, garlic should be eaten raw. One clove daily is effective, and a safe dosage for extended use. To get the most benefit, chop or crush garlic and allow to rest for 10/15 minutes, then use raw or sprinkle it over your food. This activates enzymes and releases the sulfur-containing compounds that have the most therapeutic and protective effects. To reduce the odour if it's a problem, take chlorophyll-rich foods such as parsley or wheatgrass afterwards.

Although garlic is the powerhouse of the allium family, other relatives to add to your diet include leeks, shallots, chives and of course, onions.

## CARROTS

This well-loved vegetable is packed with cancer-fighting nutrients especially the antioxidant beta-carotene, which gives it its orange colour and is believed to protect cell membranes from toxic damage and slow the growth of cancer cells. Carrots also contain other phytochemicals such as falcarinol and falcarindiol, natural pesticides that researchers believe are the reason for their cancer-fighting abilities. Scientists in England found that rats given falcarinol were less likely to develop cancerous tumours. *(11)*

In addition to beta-carotene, carrots also contain lutein and zeaxanthin, and together these three antioxidant nutrients can considerably boost eye health.

Cooked carrots supply more antioxidants than raw according to a report in the Journal of Agricultural and Food Chemistry. If you're cooking carrots, leave them whole while steaming and cut them after they're done. That reduces the loss of nutrients, including falcarinol, and gives them a sweeter taste as well. Juicing raw carrots is also an excellent way to safeguard the valuable anti-cancer nutrients.

## MUSHROOMS

When it comes to sticking to a healthy anti-cancer diet mushrooms check all the boxes. There is now a huge body of research evidence showing the protective and anti-cancer power of mushrooms.

There are a number of mushrooms known as 'medicinal mushrooms' which help the body to fight cancer and build the immune system. Among the best known are Reishi, Shiitake, Cordyceps and Maitake. These mushrooms contain a number of valuable cancer fighting and immune-boosting compounds including beta-glucans, which increase the immune system's T-cell levels; and lentinan a substance that repairs damaged DNA caused by chemo and radiation. (12)

Even the common garden button mushrooms have their benefits. These mushrooms are super dense with nutrients including zinc, potassium, copper, selenium, B-vitamins and various antioxidants. Research shows women who regularly consume button mushrooms reduce their breast cancer risks by 64%. (13. This is believed to be due to the high level of conjugated linolenic acid in these mushrooms, which is a type of fatty acid that controls the production and action of oestrogen.

Similar to button mushrooms are porcini and portobello mushrooms that are also loaded with valuable nutrients, so include these in your recipes as well. You can also take mushroom extracts in capsules that have concentrated anti-cancer compounds contained theirin.

## SEA VEGETABLES

Sea vegetables, more commonly called seaweeds contain at least ten times the mineral contents of land plants, as well as a host of other vitamins and phytochemicals. However, the most impressive component of sea vegetables is their dense concentration of fucoidan, a sulfur based polysaccharide that has shown great benefit in promoting cancer-cell death and also stimulating the immune system. Seaweeds also contain high levels of vitamins A, C and E as well as a wide range of bioflavonoids, all of which are known to prime the immune system. In addition, alginate found in sea vegetables like Nori, Kombu, Wakame and Dulse, is a natural absorbent of heavy metals and free radicals. Interestingly, the people of the Japanese island of Okinawa, who consume the highest per capita amount of Kombu, also have the highest life expectancies in the world as well as the lowest cancer death rate.

Drying the seaweed after harvesting helps to preserve the nutrients. When it's time to eat, either rehydrate it with water or use the dried form as is. Seaweeds have a pleasant salty flavour and they're so versatile to use that you can throw them into almost any dish, as you probably do with spinach. Some of the more common seaweeds that you can purchase at your supermarket or in healthfood stores include, Nori, Kombu, Dulse, Wakame, Kelp, Arame and Miso.


## BEST FOOD PREPARATION METHODS FOR VEGETABLES

While diets derived from the aforementioned vegetables already utilize a plethora of powerful health promoting and cancer prevention phytonutrients, there is a little-discussed secret that will allow you to maximize your exposure to the availability of these miracle nutrients to be more easily absorbed by your body.

The problem with vegetables is that all of their cancer-inhibiting phytonutrients are locked inside sealed compartments whose walls are composed of tough cellulose fibre. Unfortunately the human digestive system does not possess an enzyme capable of dissolving these fibrous walls. As a result, unless you can somehow break these impenetrable cell walls you'll not absorb the plant's healing nutrients.

Fortunately, there are several solutions to this dilemma, some better than others. One of them is to chew your food thoroughly. Chewing, mechanically shatters some of the plant's cell walls. The more you chew, the more they break down, but studies have shown that eating raw vegetables yields only about 30% of their nutrients, since most people do not chew vegetables until they become mush. That means most people would need to increase their vegetable intake to at least seven to eight servings per day to get any nutritional benefit. A serving is a cup of loose vegetables such as spinach or kale, or half a cup of more solid vegetables like brussels sprouts or cauliflower. A better method to break down plants tough exterior walls is by steaming or boiling. The problem with boiling is that while it easily breaks down the fibrous walls to release the plants nutrients, some will be destroyed by the intense heat while others will be lost to the water in which they are cooked.

Steaming vegetables is a better alternative because steaming avoids high heat as well as direct contact with water. Surprisingly, some vegetables contain compounds that can cause joint pain (ie peppers) and suppress thyroid function (ie broccoli, brussels sprouts, and kale) when eaten raw. Steaming destroys these harmful compounds.

The third method and in my opinion, the best is to blenderize or puree the vegetables in a food blender. No matter how much you chew raw vegetables, you will not be able to break the food down as much as a blender can.

---

### Drink Your Vegetables!

The best way to maximize your intake of anticancer nutrients is to blenderize your vegetables and drink them each day. The most potent anticancer vegetables include:

- Broccoli (especially broccoli sprouts)
- Brussels sprouts
- Cabbage
- Cauliflower
- Celery
- Kale
- Spinach
- Parsley

The biggest difference between eating raw vegetables versus blending them first, is how efficient and fast they can be digested by your body. When you blenderize vegetables, the plant's tough fibrous walls are broken down so much that they are essentially predigested. This means that your body can easily digest the vegetable puree and absorb the nutrients more effectively. It is estimated that blenderized vegetables are absorbed at a rate of 90%. This allows the body to get a much higher concentration of beneficial cancer-fighting plant compounds along with vitamins, minerals, and fibre. It also means that you can consume smaller volumes of vegetables but still get the full benefits of the recommended daily servings.

Before blenderizing vegetables, wash them thoroughly to remove any dirt or chemical residue. I'd strongly urge you to use only organic vegetables not only for their superior nutrient content and taste value, but also for the absence of chemical contaminants used to promote growth and control disease in non-organic crops. There's little excuse nowadays for not using organic food as it's very widely available in supermarkets and is not much more expensive.

Drinking a cup of blenderized vegetable juice, depending on the concentration, is equivalent to eating five to eight servings of vegetables. Most people have to develop a taste for pureed vegetables so it is best to start by diluting the mix with one third volume of purified water to two thirds vegetables. Also, some people new to this practice may not be able to tolerate the high concentration of fibre initially. So I'd advise you to start by drinking one glass of the thin blend with meals and gradually increase the volume to two full glasses (400ml) per day. After 7 to 10 days of drinking the thinner blend you can move to a more concentrated blend by adding more vegetables and less water to your blender.

The most important vegetables to blenderize include:

- Broccoli
- Brussels sprouts
- Kale
- Red cabbage

Need to be steamed first

- Savoy cabbage
- Spinach
- Cauliflower
- Celery
- Carrots
- Parsley
- Asparagus
- Coriander

# FRUIT

Fruit is one of the most delicious foods available while offering many health benefits from its treasure chest of medicinal compounds most of which are impossible to manufacture. Fruit also contains a wide range of vitamins and minerals that our bodies need to be in optimum health. Some species of fruit have health benefits that go beyond and can be helpful in dealing with one of the most vicious diseases of modern times - Cancer. One of nature's greatest bounties with its vast array of medicinal compounds and health-giving micronutrients are berries. These colourful berries such as strawberries, blueberries, raspberries, blackberries, cranberries, grapes, dark cherries and pomegranates have the greatest health value. Many of the helpful compounds found in these berries are of unique design and complexity, and have demonstrated powerful antioxidant properties, along with antibacterial, antifungal, anti-inflammatory and anti-cancer effects. In addition, berries contain higher levels of Vitamins A, C, E and B-vitamins as well as several important minerals than other fruits.

Most berries bestow a very high antioxidant protection (measured as oxygen radical absorbance capacity or ORAC units) making them some of the top ranking antioxidant foods on the planet. As well as being low in calories despite their sweetness, and also low on the glycaemic index (a measure of how they affect blood glucose levels), berries also contain a variety of phytochemicals that have been shown to prevent cancer development. These chemical compounds can also be used to treat cancer. In fact, some of these phytochemicals can stop cancer in all of its stages - initiation, promotion and progression.

Among the best anti-cancer compounds found in berries are a class of anti-oxidant-rich flavonoid compounds called, polyphenols. Research shows that these phenolic compounds offer great benefits for health due to their powerful anti-oxidant and anti-inflammatory actions.

Studies show that polyphenols can:
- Prevent cancer development
- Inhibit cancer growth and spread
- Strengthen immune function
- Kill harmful pathogens (viruses, bacteria, fungi, parasites)
- Supply energy to the body
- Interact with the microbiome to help protect the gastrointestinal tract

The most widely studied of these flavonoid compounds include quercetin, ellagic acid, anthocyanins, proanthocyanidins catechins, epicatechin, kaempferol and myricetin, which are all found in berries in various concentrations depending on the species and growing conditions.

Of the above list of compounds, one that truly stands out among them for its cancer-killing properties is ellagic acid.

## ELLAGIC ACID

Berries high in ellagic acid include, strawberries, red and black raspberries, cranberries and pomegrantes. When these berries are digested in the G.I. tract, the ellagic acid is released and the gut flora metabolizes it into compounds called urolithin A and urolithin B. These two metabolies are powerful cancer killers. In addition, they are well-absorbed into the bloodstream where they can be distributed to all organs and tissues in the body.

Studies on colon cancer have shown that black raspberries are especially effective at killing these cancer cells. It is the urolithins and especially urolithin A that is doing the killing.(14)

A number of studies have shown the cancer-destroying effects of ellagic acid, notably in breast, prostate and colon cancers. Interestingly, urolithin A from ellagic acid metabolism enhanced the effectiveness of one of the primary chemotherapy agents used against colon cancer - 5-fluorouracil (15).

Some of the major pathways by which ellagic acid stops cancer in its tracts include the following:

- Kills cancer cells by inducing apoptosis (natural cell death)
- Stops the growth and spread of cancerous tumours by protecting the cells DNA and also by strengthening the body's connective tissues.
- Stops cancer cells from multiplying by disrupting cellular division (a process called cell-cycle arrest)

# BERRIES WITH THE GREATEST HEALTH VALUE

## STRAWBERRIES

Besides being delicious, strawberries have one of the highest levels of vitamin C, a powerful antioxidant and known infection fighter. They are also a rich source of ellagic acid, anthocyanins, flavonols and some other phenolic compounds, which together pack a powerful punch. Indeed, research indicates that the blood markers from chronic inflammation can be lowered considerably by regularly eating strawberries.

In relation to strawberries cancer-inhibiting abilities, a study was carried out on a number of berries that were tested against implanted human colon, breast, oral and prostate cancers. [16] Strawberries, along with black raspberries were the most effective at killing the cancer cell lines especially the colon cancer. The flavonoid fisetin in strawberries was shown to neutralise colon, breast, cervical and prostate cancer cells.

Besides being an anticancer food, strawberries offer a host of other health benefits including cholesterol lowering and blood glucose normalizing properties. But, by far, its free radical zapping antioxidant activity is whats truly outstanding. So be sure to include lots of strawberries in your diet.


## BLUEBERRIES

Blueberries have the highest antioxidant capacity of any fruit (measured as ORAC units), due to having the highest anthocyanin content, which gives them their vivid colour. Anthocyanin compounds provide the greatest antioxidant effect of all the polyphenols. Blueberries also contain a healthy list of other beneficial flavonoids and plant compounds each unique onto themselves, but in combination offering powerful antioxidant and anti-inflammatory properties.In addition on the basic micronutrient level blueberries provide ample amounts of, vitamin C and K and the mineral manganese, an essential cofactor of the antioxidant enzyme superoxide dismutase. These nutrients, alone makes blueberries such a nutritious food.

Many of the compounds found in blueberries have been shown to significantly reduce growth of cancer by inhibiting the reproduction of cancer cells and stopping the growth of new blood vessels, which feed tumours. This makes blueberries one of the best foods, particularly in the fight against cancers of the breast, colon, small intestines and oesophagus.

In one particular study researchers examined six different berries for the anti-angiogenesis properties, and both blueberries and bilberries were the most powerful. *(17)* The blueberries inhibited two compounds that promote angiogenesis - vascular endothelial growth factor (VEGF) and TNF-alpha.

Other health benefits attributed to blueberries include robust cardiovascular health due to its cholesterol lowering properties as well as lowering blood sugar levels. In addition, blueberries can protect against the ravages of aging such as memory loss, poor coordination, weakness and general frailty. *(18)*

For optimum health, try to eat at least 1 cup of mixed berries with most emphasis on blueberries and strawberries each day.

## RASPBERRIES

The diversity of phytochemicals in raspberries is unequaled in other fruits. That's good, because while each compound by itself plays an important part in keeping the body healthy, their combined actions synergistically pack an even bigger punch. The anti-cancer benefits of raspberries is one advantage; it being attributed to their antioxidant and anti-inflammatory phytonutrients. For example, red raspberries have three times the amount of vitamin C, compared to blueberries and blackberries. Some of the cancer-inhibiting phytochemicals in raspberries include ellagic acid, ellagitannins, quercetin, gallic acid, catechins, kaempferol and salicylic acid to name but a few.

Chronic inflammation of the large intestine, called colitis is a common cause of colon cancer. Compounds that inhibit this inflammation can prevent colon cancer from developing. In one study, researchers examined the ability of red raspberries to inhibit pro-inflammatory immune cellscalled macrophageswhich were taken from colitis affected animals.*(19)* The researchers tested the crude extracts of seven berries and found that red raspberries most powerfully suppressed the inflammation of these colitis-affected animals. This was achieved mainly by reducing the release of inflammatory cytokines from the macrophages.

Red raspberries also suppressed a protein complex called NF-Kb, which drives inflammation. In addition, red raspberry extract inhibits the formation of nitric oxide in tissues. High levels of nitric oxide in the tissues as opposed to within blood vessels, (which is good), can drive cancer growth by stimulating inflammation.

Black raspberries were also found to slow the growth and even kill cancer cells of the breast and colon. Red and black raspberries with their vast array of phytonutrients bring other health benefits to those of us who consume them such as:

- Protection against diabetes
- Regulation of blood pressure
- Prevention of atherosclerosis (clogging in arteries)
- Help against obesity

So go ahead, eat them by the handful for all their nutritional goodness.

## BLACKBERRIES

Blackberries are loaded with a broad range of vitamins, minerals and flavonoid chemicals that harmoniously work together to enhance each others' medicinal properties. This humble berry is rich in vitamins A, C, E, K and B vitamins, as well as the antioxidant compound, lutein and zeaxanthin that dampen down inflammation, which plays a major role in cancer development. Minerals such as copper, magnesium, manganese and potassium are also found in this berry.

Blackberries are also a rich source of phenolic compounds such as ellagic acid, anthocyanins, quercetin, catechins, kaempferol, gallic acid, cyanidins, myricetin and salicylic acid. These antioxidant compounds quench damaging free radicals and so protect against degenerative disease including cancer.

Of the cyanidin compounds found in blackberries, cyanidin 3-glucoside in particular has been found to have chemo-protective activity [20].

Ellagic acid, another potent cancer inhibitor and myricetin with its antioxidant actions are both ingredients in blackberries. Together these three compounds exert a powerful anti-cancer effect, way more so than any one of them alone. Make sure you add this tasty fruit to your berry mix.

## CRANBERRIES

Among the best anti-cancer fruits are cranberries, which are rich in the polyphenols. The primary phenolic compound that is abundant in cranberries and which gives them their bright red colour is anthocyanins. These anthocyanins, along with ellagic acid, quercetin and other polyphenols that are present in cranberries minimize the damaging effects of free radicals on the cells DNA, which can cause cancer. Vitamin C is another antioxidant that helps prevent cancer and is found in abundance in this delicious fruit.

Many studies demonstrate a variety of health benefits provided by cranberries, from being a well-known urinary tract antiseptic to a protector against cancer, particularly breast cancer, due in part to its potent antioxidant polyphenols.

One study in particular listed several diseases cranberries can protect against including some cancers *(21)*. Cranberry extract was able to inhibit the growth and spread of cancer cells and also induce natural cell death (apoptosis) in some cancer cell lines.

Fresh cranberries contain the most antioxidants, dried cranberries run a close second while cranberry juice contains the least amount. If buying cranberry juice make sure that it is 100% juice and not a cranberry drink, which is usually laced with sugar.

## GRAPES

Grapes contain powerful flavonoid compounds that can inhibit cancer development. There is a natural phenolic compound contained in the skin of grapes called resveratrol and is found in abundance in dark red and black grapes. It has been clinically proven that the treatment of colon cancer cells with resveratrol significantly reduces the activity of an enzyme called ornithne decarboxylase. This enzyme is the culprit in the growth of cancer cells. The less of this in your body the better. Resveratrol also has a good reputation for lowering "bad" cholesterol and preventing clogging in artery walls, thereby preventing cardiovascular disease and neurological conditions such as alzheimer's. Grapes are also a rich source of anthocyanins, catechins and ellagic acid, three powerful flavonoids that slow the growth of cancer tumours by reducing inflammation and by blocking enzymes needed by cancer cells. In addition, grapes are rich in micronutrients like copper and magnanese, an essential co-factor of the antioxidant enzyme superoxide dismutase.

People who regularly eat grapes reduce the risk of developing cancer, especially of the colon, breast and prostate. Make sure to eat the entire grape, seeds and all.

## POMEGRANATE

With over 100 different polyphenols, including flavonoids, punicalagins, anthocyanins and ellagic acid pomegranate juice tops the list of "healthiest juices" for antioxidant activity, ahead of grape juice, blueberry juice, and acai juice. Refreshing, colourful and tangy, pomegranate and pomegranate juice is not only delicious but a valuable weapon against cancer.

All parts of the pomegranate plant, including the fruit, peel and seeds, are rich in compounds that protect against chemical and physical threats to our cells. These compounds include several families of polyphenols called tannins and flavonoids, which give it its vivid scarlet colour.

For years, scientists have been studying these bioactive compounds for their anti-cancer benefits. Pomegranate extracts help combat cancer in several of the stages of tumour development. These mechanisms include protecting DNA from damage, inhibiting excessive cell growth, promoting natural cancer cell death by apoptosis, and preventing cancer from spreading. *(22, 23, 24)*

## A POTENT CANCER BLOCKER

Research shows that pomegranate extracts have the unique ability to promote the production of a protective enzyme called paraoxonase - 1 (PON-1), which blocks oxidative damage and inflammation that can cause DNA mutations which trigger cancer development. *(25)* In fact, people with cancer have been found in many studies to have low levels of PON-1, therefore if we consume pomegranates, we'll help restore and promote PON-1 activity which will in turn block cancer development at its earliest stages.

Overall pomegranate food and it's extracts have shown great promise in preventing the growth and spread of six common types of cancer cells: breast, prostate, lung, colon, skin and liver cell cancers.(26)

Pomegranate extracts, are available in powder and capsule form with the recommended dosage been between 500mg and 1500mg daily. You can also drink pomegranate juice just make sure it is 100% pure and not a cocktail or a blend with added sugars. Most experts recommend drinking between 200 and 300 ml of pomegranate juice per day.

## TOMATOES

Technically speaking tomatoes are a fruit and they are also the epitome of a cancer-fighting superfood. Not only do tomatoes contain lycopene, an antioxidant phytochemical that gives them their bright red colour, they are also a good source of vitamins A, C and E; all enemies of cancer-friendly free radicals. By now you know a lot about the power of antioxidants and especially bioflavonoids, with their ability to neutralize harmful free radicals in the body. Well lycopene shows up in a big way in tomatoes. This powerful antioxidant flavonoid compound has the ability to protect cells from damage and kill those that aren't growing properly. Several studies suggest that a lycopene-rich diet is connected to a reduced risk of prostate cancer. In laboratory tests lycopene has also stopped other types of cancer cells from growing, including breast, and lung. It is speculated that lycopene stops the growth of tumours by interfering with cancer cell growth and also through boosting the immune system. Lycopene also plays a part in lowering cholesterol and triglycereds in the bloodstream and so protecting against heart disease.

The secret to getting the full health benefits of tomatoes lies in the preparation. Unlike other fruits that are best eaten raw, eating cooked tomatoes makes the cancer-fighting lycopene more available to your body because heat breaks down the plant's cell walls.

So, roasting tomatoes in the oven, drinking tomato soup and eating canned tomatoes gives you much higher concentrations of lycopene than fresh. It is recommended you consume 25-40 mgs of lycopene daily for optimum benefits, this equates to roughly one large tomato per day.

## AVOCADO

Many people think avocados are vegetables, but in reality they are fruit and are one of the best foods on the planet that you can eat. Not only are they a great source of healthy mono-unsaturated fats; the kind that helps you lose weight while keeping your cholesterol levels in the healthy range and so, lowering your risk of heart disease; they are also jam-packed with over twenty vitamins and minerals that provide many health benefits, including protection against cancer.

For instance, avocados have a high content of vitamin C, a powerful antioxidant that neutralizes free radicals, which can otherwise damage the cell's DNA and potentially lead to cancer formation. In addition, carotenoids found in avocados (beta-carotene, alfa-carotene and zeaxanthin) help prevent cancer of the skin, breast, prostate and oesophagus. Also, the abundance of the fat-soluble vitamins A, E and K found in avocados can drastically reduce the incidence of cancer, especially breast cancer. Avocados also contain glutathione, an antioxidant that protects the body's cells from cancer development and the dangerous effects of free-radical damage.

Some studies have shown that phytochemicals in avocados help inhibit cancer cell division through a process called cell-cycle arrest. They also induce apoptosis (programmed cell death) in precancerous and cancer cell lines.(27)

And more recently, a new study reveals more of avocados' cancer killing weapons. Researchers in Canada have found a fat molecule in avocado that fights a virulent form of leukaemia called Acute Myeloid Leukaemia (AML). The compound is called avocatin B. It targets and kills AML stem cells. These are the cells that drive the cancer by constantly churning out cancerous daughter cells. And unlike chemotherapy drugs, avocatin B seems to help preserve the healthy cells.(28)

Many other studies have also touted avocado a useful cancer-fighting food. The Journal of Nutrition and Cancer published the results of a study claiming that the phytochemicals in avocados are so powerful that they could prevent the use of chemotherapy in people suffering from oral cancer. (29)

Other health benefits gained from eating avocados include better weight control, protection from heart disease and diabetes, lowering of inflammation in the body, improved digestion, better cognitive functions and mental health, better vision and better skin and hair.

So, adding more avocado to your diet is a 'no-brainer' because not only might it prevent you from getting cancer in the first place, it has been clearly shown to destroy cancer directly. You should aim to eat at least half an avocado added to your salad each day, or use it to give a creamy touch to your smoothies. You could also make a batch of guacamole to serve with snacks or dinner. If you want to give an interesting touch to your dishes, try cooking with some avocado oil, or try using a bit of avocado oil in place of olive oil for salad dressings or drizzled on your wild salmon.

---

### GOOD ADVICE ✓

The more colourful the fruit or vegetable, the higher its antioxidant count is likely to be. Green leafy vegetables like spinach are much more healthful than iceberg lettuce – that stable of your typical salad that has little nutritional value. Blueberries, strawberries, and raspberries are antioxidant rich. So take colour into consideration when planning your meal.

---

---
**Chapter 6**
---

# Nutritional Supplementation in the fight against Cancer

Two time Nobel Prize winner Dr. Linus Pauling declared,
*"Nearly all disease can be traced to a nutritional deficiency".*

Research has demonstrated that our modern-day diet is usually not sufficient to supply all the nutrients necessary for overall good health. As a consequence nutrient deficiencies which are prevalent today, can contribute to overall weakening of the body and its immune defences making a person more vulnerable to cancer.

Our bodies require a range of nutrients including vitamins and minerals to fulfil the hundreds of thousands of biochemical reactions that keep us healthy. If there are deficiencies in one or more of these nutrients at the appropriate level deemed necessary for health, the body will malfunction and overtime will develop some form of disease including cancer. In fact, years of research has made it increasingly clear that deficiencies in certain vitamins and minerals are linked to increased cancer risk.

When it comes to diet and cancer, conventional oncologists genuinely know very little about nutrition so they rarely make any dietary recommendations. Even worse, some cancer doctors tell patients there is no relationship between their diet and cancer. The truth is your diet along with specific nutrient supplementation can make all the difference between recovering or succumbing to this deadly disease.

> Most of my cancer clients have already received chemotherapy and radiation, so I must not only treat the cancer, but also the side effects of those orthodox treatments. Many people who have had chemotherapy suffer from nutritional deficiencies, since their oncologists do not pay close attention to this issue.

And when it comes to supplements, oncologists tend to be downright hostile, believing that vitamins, minerals and herbs will negatively interfere with conventional treatments or have no benefit. Nothing could be further from the truth. There is now a substantial body of research showing that vitamins and minerals do not interfere with chemotherapy or radiation. Instead, these micronutrients have been shown to increase survival times, kill cancer cells, make chemo and radiation more effective and even minimise the horrendous side effects of both treatments.

Let me quote from a recent study reported in the Journal of Biophotonics that shows that nutrients not only do not interfere with chemotherapy drugs, they actually make them more effective, while also reducing the side effects of chemotherapy.

To do the experiment, researchers treated HeLa cells with a chemotherapy drug camptothecin. Camptothecin is a potent anticancer drug which is known to kill cervical cancer cells. HeLa cells are an immortal cancer cell line routinely used in scientific research. They treated some of the cells with camptothecin only, and they treated other cells with camptothecin plus the antioxidant vitamin E. So, what happened?

According to the researchers: "We conclusively prove that presence of vitamin E at 100uM concentration shows promising antioxidant activity and displays no modulatory role on camptothecin induced effect, thereby causing no possible hindrance with the efficacy of the drug".[1] In addition, they stated, "vitamin E may prove beneficial to alleviate chemotherapy associated side-effects in patients."

So, if you are getting chemotherapy, let me very strongly suggest that you not only consult with an oncologist open to the use of nutrient supplementation in conjunction with chemo and radiation, but that you also consult with a therapist well-versed in the use of nutrients and other natural treatments.

Dr. Charles Simone an oncologist who has written several books and scientific papers about the hundreds of studies involving thousands of patients shows that a broad range of nutritional supplements, including antioxidants, protects you from the ravages of chemo drugs and radiotherapy while at the same time improving their outcomes.[2]

Upon reviewing these studies, he found that those who took supplements did not compromise their cancer therapy or end up with worse results. Furthermore, he found that supplements actually:

- Protected patients from some of chemo's and radiation's worst side effects
- Enhanced chemo and radiation effectiveness
- Protected healthy cells from the damaging effects of chemo and radiation
- Improved patients overall health
- Lengthened survival times

I'm often asked by clients and friends whether nutritional supplements are really needed if one is eating a balanced diet. My answer is that if we lived in an ideal world where no environmental pollutants existed and our food had perfect composition, then we would be eating a perfect disease-thwarting diet and so, there would be no need for supplements.

This idealistic scenario may have been possible a few hundred years ago, before the advent of the Industrial Age and when food was grown organically on fertile soil. The land was not stripped of its nutrients through any refining and packaging process, and so contained all the nutrients that nature intended.

Today however, the choice to eat a nutritionally balanced diet is no longer within our control. The foods we now eat are desperately lacking in essential vitamins and minerals as a result of them being stripped of much of their nutrient content through over-processing and refining techniques. In addition, due to intensive farming practices our soils have become depleted of many minerals essential for human health.

While modern agriculture adds nitrogen (N) phosphorus (P) and potassium (K) to the soil, which are the only minerals plants require for growth the remaining 60 minerals that are found in the human body are not added to the soil; thus are found in ever-diminishing amounts in our diet and bodies. This is not good as there are some crucial minerals involved in cancer prevention and reversal such as selenium, zinc, magnesium, chromium and iodine.

Also, the food crops growing on these depleted soils are loaded with residues of fungicides, herbicides, pesticides, along with other chemical and environmental pollutants that can play havoc with our bodies. In addition, the majority of fruits and vegetables are either sprayed or dipped in more chemicals at harvest time and then left in cold storage for long periods, further depleting their nutrient content. For example; frozen vegetables lose about a third of their vitamins during the freezing process. Fruits can lose 50% of their vitamin C within one day of harvest. On top of that most fruits are picked while still unripe and before they have time to manufacture the majority of their vitamins. Consequently, most food that arrives on our tables has very little in the way of vitamins, minerals, or other phytonutrients essential to human health.

While a cumulative lack of these essential vitamins and minerals can contribute to the onset of chronic conditions including cancer, the correct fortification with these missing nutrients can start to reverse such conditions. When you consider that vitamins and minerals function are to "drive" the biochemical and electrical circuitry of the body, and that every bodily function totally depends on energy-producing (ATP) chemical reactions that are used by our cells to carry out their life-sustaining metabolic functions. This finely-tuned orchestra of biochemical activity depends on the availability of specific vitamins and minerals; and without adequate amounts of these nutrients, together with the requisite macro-nutrients of carbs, protein and fats in our diet, then energy is reduced at the cellular level, health and vitality diminishes and illness will occur.

## POSITIVE EVIDENCE FOR THE VALUE OF SUPPLEMENTS IN REVERSING CANCER

For decades, many doctors discouraged cancer patients from taking supplements. That has changed. Today, even mainstream cancer clinics recognize the growing evidence that supplements effectively fight cancer. Study after study shows that supplements not only prevent and treat cancer, they can ease the side effects of chemo and radiations. And they can help patients recover faster after surgery.

It's no longer a question of whether supplements work, but which ones work best. Saying that, I'm not going to tell you that simply taking a supplement will cure your cancer because that's generally just not true. But what supplements can do is give you a big health boost and send your survival odds skyrocketing. You will have better results because supplements attack cancer in ways that chemotherapy and radiation can't.

## MORE ANTIOXIDANTS MEANS LESS CANCER

An antioxidant is a substance such as vitamin C, vitamin E, or beta-cartene that protects body cells from the damaging effects of oxidation. Oxidation damages cells including their DNA which can lead to the development of diseases including cancer. Antioxidants play an important role in preventing such damage and also, in finding and repairing damaged cells, as well as boosting your immune system.

Let's look now at the following three studies where cancer patients and healthy people alike were taking simple antioxidants versus none and see the difference.

- In an Italian study carried out between 1991 and 1994, the dietary habits of 2,569 women aged between 20-74 yrs with breast cancer were compared to an equal number of women in the same age range without cancer. *(3)* Researchers found that the women with cancer had significantly lower intakes of the antioxidants beta-carotene, Vitamin E and calcium than the cancer-free women.

- The Americans conducted a five-year study of 38,000 Chinese people who took a daily antioxidant combination of beta-carotene, vitamin E and the mineral selenium. The study, which finished in 1993 found that these people had a 13% less chance of developing cancer and of those who did get cancer a 21% less chance of dying from it compared to the general population who took no anti-oxidant supplements. *(4)*

- The French conducted a 7 ½ year study (Su. Vi. Max study) on 13,000 people which was completed in 2004. All participants took a single daily capsule of either a low dose antioxidant combination (Vitamins C, E, beta-carotene, selenium and zinc) or a placebo dummy pill. The researchers concluded that the antioxidant supplements lowered the incidence of cancer in those men who initially had a lower baseline status of antioxidants, especially beta-carotene. *(5)*

## A BRIEF REVIEW OF SPECIFIC MICRO-NUTRIENTS IN REVERSING CANCER:

## VITAMIN D

People usually think of vitamin D as a nutrient we need for our bones. And we do. However, it is also a real cancer-fighting superstar. Studies have shown that this vital vitamin can help cut your cancer risk and support your recovery after a diagnosis. In general people who have higher levels of vitamin D have significantly lower rates of all cancers by as much as 50% to 75%. That's significant! *(6)*

Vitamin D deficiency has also been linked to other conditions including, osteoporosis, rheumatoid arthritis, diabetes, heart disease, multiple sclerosis and inflammatory bowel disease. (7) Scaremongering about the negative effects of sunshine, coupled with indoor lifestyles and gloomy weather have led to widespread deficiency of this essential nutrient. According to some estimates, nearly 40% of otherwise healthy young adults don't have enough. In people with health problems, nearly 60% are low in vitamin D in the USA. Here in Europe these percentages are higher. (8) And maybe, that's one possible reason for the increase in cancers we see today.

There are a number of mechanisms by which vitamin D reduces the risk of cancer:

For starters, it helps us absorb calcium. And calcium plays an important role in healthy cell differentiation. It is also essential in activating the T-cells in the immune systemwhich can then chase down rogue cancer cells. What's more vitamin D affects other areas that can increase cancer risks. For instance it helps regulate insulin resistance (cancer is a sugar feeder); It lowers blood inflammatory markers (cancer grows and spreads in an inflammatory environment) it stops angiogenesis (the growth of blood vessels that feed a tumour), it reduces metastastis and proliferation in existing cancer; and increases apoptosis (programmed cell death). It does this by helping the body to make a crucial protein that induces cancer cell death. (9)

More than 60 studies have found that high levels of Vitamin D are associated with a lower risk of certain cancers including breast, ovarian, prostate, colon and lung. (10)

It is well known that vitamin D deficiency puts women at a higher risk of breast cancer. (11) This fact has prompted Professor Hollick from Harvard Medical School to state that there would be 25% less women dying from breast cancer if they took adequate daily levels of vitamin D. This bold statement deserves credence as a 2014 report in the Journal Anti-Cancer Research found that breast cancer survivors with the highest vitamin D levels had HALF the death rate of those with low levels. (12)

Yet another study showed that women who spent a lot of time in the sunshine (which is what creates vitamin D) had up to 45% less cancers than those who didn't sunbathe. Bottom line: get more 'safe' sun and find a good supplement of absorbable vitamin D. The form of vitamin D which you need is D3 (cholecalciferal) and not the synthetic form D2 (eogocalciferal). Vitamin D3 is produced from UVB rays in sunlight and is also found is high amounts in wild salmon, mackerel, tuna, cod liver oil, eggs, mushrooms and beef.

All recent reports suggest 4,000 to 5,000 IUs per day as the correct dosage for cancer patients. For healthy people a daily intake of 1,000 to 2,000 IUs is sufficient to help protect against cancer.

In men, the prostate gland also needs Vitamin D. In one study using vitamin D3 supplements, 50% of patients with prostate cancer had reduced or maintained their PSA level. (13) This was at a dosage of just 2,000IUs per day. But like I suggested already and as some experts say, you may need between 4,000 and up to 10,000 IU per day. Just imagine what kind of results that could produce.


# VITAMIN C

Vitamin C has many functions in the body's metabolism, many of them directly related to either preventing and/or recovering from cancer. Here is a list of the major roles Vitamin C plays in the body:

- It is a potent antioxidant preventing free radical damage to cells and tissues

- It supports optimal immune function to protect against infections and cancer

- It is involved in the synthesis of collagen and elastin; fibres that make up connective tissue, which is the 'glue' that keeps our body together

- It is known to stimulate the production of a compound that inhibits the release of hyaluronidase, an enzyme that cancer cells produce as a means to 'eat their way through the body's connective tissue.'

- It is a general detoxifier as it can bind with chemical pollutants to render them safe

- It converts cholesterol into bile for its elimination in the bowels

- It is a regulator of insulin to better control blood sugar levels

- Vitamin C is also involved in the production of adrenaline for energy and serotonin for thought and calmness. It is also important for the health of bone, cartilage, gums and teeth, and also plays a very important role in iron absorption, thus impacting overall body health in many critical ways.

Let's look at how Vitamin C can help cancer patients in more detail. Studies in the 1970's and 1980's conducted by Nobel Prize winner and veteran pioneer Vitamin C researcher, Linus Pauling suggest that very large doses of Vitamin C taken both intravenously and orally is preferentially toxic to cancer cells. Pauling, along with his medical collaborator Dr. Ewan Cameron published several studies on the beneficial response of cancer patients to large doses of supplemental vitamin C as an adjunct treatment to chemotherapy and radiation. They found repeatedly that benefits ranged from a complete cessation of pain with an increased sense of well-being, an earlier discharge from hospital and an increased survival time for terminal patients to rare but complete remissions of some cancers. Pauling found that vitamin C infusions helped terminally ill cancer patients live about four times longer than similar patients not given vitamin C.

Now I'm of the opinion that had Pauling given his cancer patients other natural substances as outlined in this book, along with the vitamin C protocol he prescribed, he would have had a near 100% success rate, but as a doctor, he was probably not aware of the miraculous healing powers of these natural compounds, as such information is not taught at medical school.

Usually the body keeps a tight rein on vitamin C levels in the blood. Pauling knew that only high concentrations of ascorbic acid (i.e. Vitamin C) in blood serum were effective in killing cancer. These levels could not be achieved by the oral route only. So Pauling found that the body's mechanism could be bypassed if the vitamin was injected straight into the bloodstream instead of passing through the digestive system. When this is done it releases the powerful anti-cancer potential of the vitamin.

But despite these positive outcomes, Pauling's strident critics and peers from the cancer establishment refused to believe that an inexpensive vitamin C could cure cancer.

One Charles Moertel, MD, of the Mayo Clinic allegedly followed the Pauling protocol and found no benefit with vitamin C *(14)* in terminal colon cancer patients. But the problem was, Moertel did not follow Pauling's protocol: The Mayo studies used only oral vitamin C whereas Pauling used IV vitamin C as well as oral. The intravenous route will result in far higher blood levels of Vitamin C, which is necessary to kill cancer.

This isn't to say that taking vitamin C orally is of no beneficial effect. To the contrary, high-dose oral intake of vitamin C at tapered doses can help maximise your body's immune system, strengthen connective tissue and aid in tissue repair. But, when it comes to effectively treating cancer, intravenous administration is the only way to go.

Linus Pauling offered several reasons why Moertel and subsequent studies had not found such positive results. First, the dosages were too low; second, the supplements were discontinued prematurely; third, patients who had been heavily pre-treated with chemotherapy drugs and radiation therapy were damaged beyond the point of recovery. There is a biological limit that needs to be recognised. Once a patient passes that limitthey are unlikely to respond to even the best of therapies.

In relation to vitamin C curing cancer, Pauling never made such claims, he only suggested high doses of vitamin C in concert with oncology therapies would augment cancer outcome. He later went on to explain the reasons why vitamin C may improve outcome in cancer treatment including:

- The increased need for vitamin C in cancer patients
- The ability of vitamin C to hinder cancer cells breaking down connective tissue as a means to spread;

- The ability of vitamin C to help 'wall off' or encapsulate tumours
- The role of vitamin C in immune attack on cancers
- The role of vitamin C in detoxification and in hormonal balance *(15)*

All these positive effects can be obtained by supplementation of either oral or injectable vitamin C. Only the injectable vitamin C can raise the blood serum to the required levels to directly kill cancer cells.

The basis of vitamin C's cancer-fighting ability can be attributed in large part to its antioxidant properties and alsoits immune function.

## VITAMIN C's PROPERTY AS AN ANTIOXIDANT

One of the explanations why vitamin C kills cancer cells but not healthy cells lies in the fact that vitamin C generates large amounts of hydrogen peroxide ($H_2O_2$), a potent free radical, which is neutralized in healthy cells by the enzyme catalase. *(16)* Cancer cells do not have this enzyme to protect them and so are vulnerable to hydrogen peroxide. This chemical compound forms in the spaces between cancer cells, damaging membranes, upsetting metabolism and scrambling DNA. Any cancer cells that are not immediately killed are rendered more vulnerable to the anti-cancer effects of chemotherapy and radiation.

Vitamin C is also easily absorbed by cancer cells, because its chemical structure is similar to the glucose molecule (cancer's preferred food). Because cancer cells have a voracious appetite for glucose they inadvertently take in a lot of vitamin C as well. As a consequence of the faulty metabolism that occurs inside the cancer cells' mitochondria, these cells produce high levels of "redox-active" iron molecules. These molecules react with vitamin C to form more hydrogen peroxide, that drives cancer cell death by damaging the cells DNA and structure *(17)*.

## VITAMIN C's ROLE IN THE MAINTENANCE OF A HEALTHY IMMUNE SYSTEM

The significant role that vitamin C plays in the proper functioning of the immune system is now well documented. Not only is vitamin C present in high concentrations in immune cells such as natural killer (NK) cells, which seek out and destroy cancer cells, it has also been shown to be necessary for these cells proper functioning.*(18)*

Vitamin C is also known to be consumed in the body at much higher rates in the presence of infection. Immune system functioning works not only to prevent and fight infections; help the body's tissue heal after injury (e.g. surgery) but also works to combat cancer. The immune systems role in fighting cancer is a versatile and multifaceted one, involved in not only fighting cancer, but also preventing it from taking hold in the first place. *(19)*

The important role that vitamin C plays in supporting healthy immune function therefore highlights the important function of vitamin C as an anti-cancer agent.

In addition to its own anti-cancer properties, vitamin C has also been shown to increase the effectiveness of certain chemotherapy agents in fighting cancer. Examples include cisplatin, paclitaxel, dacarbazine and doxorubicin, in addition to the anti-oestrogen agent Tamoxifen that is used in treating breast cancer. *(20, 21)*

## Forms of Vitamin C

Vitamin C comes in various forms. The type most commonly sold is ascorbic acid, which in higher doses can produce acid overload and is less well-absorbed than ascorbate. The best type is magnesium ascorbate, but that is hard to find.

Most supplements are calcium ascorbate or a mixture of magnesium and calcium ascorbate. Above a dose of 500mg, most ascorbate absorption falls rapidly. A novel form that greatly increases the absorption of vitamin C is called Lypo-Spheric Vitamin C. It comes as a powdered form in small packets of 1,000mg.

Another form is ascorbyl palmitate, which unlike the other forms of vitamin C is fat-soluble – meaning it accumulates in the fatty parts of the cell. You can take these two forms together. Again, to reduce the risk of excess iron absorption, take your vitamin C between meals. The maintenance dose is 1,000mg four times a day.

## Dosage:

Vitamin C is usually started at between 4-6 grams a day in divided oral doses. This daily dosage is then increased until bowel tolerance is attained. That's when you start to get very loose bowels including diarrhoea. The dosage is then reduced to just below that level and maintained for several months and preferably lifelong.

As you increase your vitamin C dose, the percentage that is absorbed into your bloodstream goes down. To help overcome this, the mineral-bound vitamins C such as calcium ascorbate or magnesium ascorbate will provide a more prolonged and sustained blood level of ascorbate. As vitamin C has a short half-life of only 2 hours in the human body it is best to take it in divided doses throughout the day. There is also a more expensive liposomal vitamin C that wraps the vitamin in small balloons of fat as happens under normal digestion. This delivers far higher blood levels. Also, one gram of liposomal vitamin C is equivalent to 10 grams of the mineral bound ascorbate and without the side effects.

# VITAMIN E

You may know that Vitamin E plays an important role in maintaining healthy skin and vision, but extensive research indicates it can do much more than that. It has been shown to protect the body from a plethora of diseases such as arthritis, heart disease, diabetes, heart, lung and kidney disease and also cancer. [22]

Natural vitamin E is a fat-soluble vitamin that is found mostly in the main cell membranes around cells, and the membranes that encase various organelles such as mitochondria and the cellnucleus within the cell. One of the main functions of vitamin E is to protect these membranes from damage by destructive free radicals and lipid peroxidation metabolites, rendering them harmless before they get a chance to harm DNA, therefore preventing mutations and tumour growth.

Because vitamin E is a potent antioxidant (along with vitamin C), most conventional oncologists tend to assume that since these nutrients are antioxidants, and chemotherapy and radiation work by generating pro-oxidants to kill cancer cells, therefore these vitamins reduce the efficiency of chemo and radiation in cancer patients. Nothing could be further from the truth. Vitamin E has been shown to boost the effectiveness of chemotherapy drugs on tumours, as well as protecting healthy cells against the toxic effects of such agents and radiation. *(23)*

So vitamin E is a valuable and essential ally for both the cancer patient and the oncologist, especially considering the fact that a deficiency of vitamin E has been associated with many cancers especially prostate, colon and lung cancers *(22)*

Even though its name makes it sound like a single substance, vitamin E is actually a mixture of eight related compounds, four called tocopherols and four called tocotrienols. These compounds are classified as alpha beta, gamma and delta for each category. As increasing information has become available about these forms of vitamin E, more and more of them are understood to have unique functions. Until recently the vast majority of research had been directed at the tocopherol forms of Vitamin E, but newer research has discovered that the tocotrienols have a more potent antioxidant effect as well as inhibiting cancer growth and spread.

In recent research tocotrienols have displayed very impressive cancer-inhibiting properties against a wide variety of cancers including the more deadly forms such as pancreatic cancer *(24)* and brain cancers *(25)*. But the most striking finding is that tocotrienols powerfully inhibit cancer spread (metastasis) which is what makes cancer deadly. They do so by reducing the inflammation around the tumour site, which in turn reduces angiogenesis - the formation of new blood vessels that feed tumours.

Studies have shown that beta, delta and gamma forms of tocotrienols have very potent anti-angiogenic activity.*(26)* These tocotrienol subtypes also inhibit cancer growth and spread by a number of other mechanisms including:

- Inhibition of factors that stimulate angiogenesis

- Inhibition of oncogene expression (genes that promote cancer development)
- Activation of tumour killer genes
- Regulation and enhancement of immune response to cancer [27, 28]

In previous research it was shown that deficiencies in vitamin E result in an increase in lipid peroxidation (pro-oxidants) that decrease energy production (due to mitochondriol membrane damage); increase mutations in the DNA, and alters the normal transport mechanisms in the cell membrane [29]

This subtle ongoing damage eventually translates into poor immune function, cognitive deterioration and cardiovascular disease and cancer. A recent meta-analysis of 11 studies concluded that patients with low blood concentrations of vitamin E had a higher risk of colorectal cancer. [30]

Other studies assessing the anti-cancer potential of vitamin E found that:
- Vitamin E supplements (200-400 mg) for three months, reversed fibrocystic breast disease (a major risk factor for breast cancer) in 22 out of 26 women [31]
- The tocotrienols in vitamin E have been shown to powerfully stimulate the death of breast cancer cells including the most aggressive breast cancers in cultures[32]
- Vitamin E reduces lung cancer risk by up to 53% [33]
- Gamma-tocotrienol, one of the vitamin E constituents may decrease prostate tumour formation by 75% [34]

## VITAMIN E MINIMISES DAMAGE FROM CHEMOTHERAPY AND RADIATION TREATMENT

Vitamin E helps these toxic treatments to distinguish between healthy and cancerous cells. What makes vitamin E so beneficial is that it easily enters healthy cells where it can protect them from the prooxidant generating chemo drugs and radiation treatments. Vitamin E, on the other hand, is not well absorbed or needed by cancer cells, since they are anaerobic (don't use oxygen) and haven't the mechanisms to utilize antioxidants to their benefit. Because of this weakness, chemotherapy and radiation can be made much more selectively toxic to the cancer cells, while vitamin E protects healthy cells.

## FOODS WITH VITAMIN E

Vitamin E can easily be obtained from a healthy diet, so before considering a supplement, consider including more vitamin E rich foods in your diet. Foods are the ideal source of vitamin E as all eight vitamin E compounds are naturally available. Vitamin E is synthesized by plants and the highest amounts are found in plant oil such as wheat germ oil, palm oil and rice bran oil. Other foods that contain generous amounts of vitamin E include:

- Sunflower seeds
- Almonds
- Hazelnuts
- Sesame
- Linseed
- high fat / oil rich plants such as olives and avocados
- Mango
- Butternut squash
- Leafy greens
- Fatty fish

## Daily anti-cancer dosage

Levels of vitamin E have been declining in foods, primarily because of over processing. This has led to widespread deficiency among the populace (35) where it is estimated that only a fifth of the world's population are receiving the recommended vitamin E intake.

Since vitamin E is fat-soluble, taking it with a fatty meal helps increase its absorption. Make sure you ever only take a totally natural vitamin E that includes all the tocopherols and tocotrienols, and has a strength of 400 iu's per capsule. Most commercially available vitamin E supplements are derived from petrochemicals and have no health benefits. They are labelled as DL-alpha-tocopherol or d-alpha-tocopherol acetate. In fact, this is the form most commonly used when investigating the health effects of vitamin E. Plus, it has been shown to have no anti-cancer activity as it interferes with the beneficial natural vitamin E and in high enough doses, or taking it long term may increase the risk of death. (36)

On the other hand, studies done on the natural form of vitamin E (ie the mixture of four tocopherols and four tocotrienols) have consistently demonstrated excellent anti-cancer activity, immune boosting effects, powerful anti-inflammatory effects and powerful antioxidanteffects. So, if you opt for a supplement (and I recommend you do in conjunction with a good diet) look for a foods based supplement that has a balance of all eight types of vitamin E (four tocopherols and four tocotrienols.)

## BETA-CAROTENE AND VITAMIN A

Beta-Carotene, classified as a carotenoid is a strongly coloured red-orange pigment abundant in most fruits and vegetables. Within the body, it is converted to vitamin A in concert with the body's own needs for the vitamin.

Beta-carotene, along with other carotenoids (alpha-carotene, lutein, lycopene, zeascanthin and others) have been thoroughly reviewed regarding their role in cancer and it has been found that "carotenoids exert an important influence in modulating the actions of carcinogens." (37)

Beta-carotene and many other carotenoids have strong anti-oxidant activity; protecting the body from damaging free radicals and blocking the proliferation of cancer cells. Beta-carotene has been shown to affect the cancer process in a number of ways:

- Maintains proper cell-to-cell communication. Cells communicate via a telegraph system of charged ions floating in and out of cell membrane pores. This intercellular communication helps to maintain cooperation and coordination between cells. Without beta-carotene and/or vitamin A, this telegraph system becomes distorted and cancer can arise. *(38)*

- Enhances the activity of natural killer (NK) cells and other immune cells against tumours. *(39)*

- It's a potent antioxidant, which protects immune cells in their battle against cancer

- Protects the DNA against the damaging effects of free radicals and carcinogens

- Once cancer has been initiated, beta-carotene inhibits the next developmental stage in the cancer process *(40)*

The principle dietary source of beta-carotene is fruit and vegetables such as carrots, pumpkin, sweet potato, apricots, spinach and kale. Since beta-carotene is only one of the many beneficial carotenoids, it is important to eat a wide variety of fresh fruit and vegetables to obtain a full spectrum of these important nutrients in your diet. All of these carotenoids work together in synergy, so taking high doses of any one of them in isolation could offset the activities of the others. For this reason it may be preferable to supplement with a mixed carotenoid complex containing a mixture of alpha and beta-carotene, lycopene, lutein, zeaxanthin, canthoxanthin and others. Take 25,000 iu daily.

# VITAMIN A

Vitamin A is a fat-soluble vitamin that has powerful antioxidant properties. It plays a critical role in a wide range of biological processes in the body including cell division and differentiation, immune regulation, maintenance of epithelial tissue, and like all good anti-oxidants, it's also excellent at reducing inflammation by fighting damaging free radicals.

Vitamin A was the first micronutrient to be recognised for its role in preventing cancer. A study conducted in 1926 where rats fed on a diet low in vitamin A developed stomach cancer. In 1941, a focused study involving humans with the same cancer found they had low plasma (blood) levels of vitamin A. Since that time there has been numerous studies linking low Vitamin A levels with cancers of the lung, breast, prostate and gastrointestinal tract.

Vitamin A which exists primarily in the form of retinol is a key nutrient in human nutrition whose many functions relate either directly or indirectly to the cancer patient. Because of its central role in a wide range of biological processes including regulation of cell growth and cell differentiation, several studies have examined the association of this vitamin and various types of cancer. These accumulated studies have prompted the National Institute of Health in America to state that: "Dietary intake studies suggest an association between diets rich in beta-carotene and vitamin A and a lower risk of many types of cancer. A higher intake of green and yellow vegetables or other food sources of beta-carotene and/or vitamin A may decrease the risk of lung cancer." *(41)*

A prospective cohort study of over 82,000 people, published in the American Journal of Clinical Nutrition in 2007 showed that high intakes of vitamin A reduced the risk of stomach cancer by 50% *(42)*

In general, most of the research into vitamin A seems to indicate its greatest benefit is in preventing cancers or recurrences of cancer. A drug analog of vitamin A (all trans retinoic acid) has become a near cure-all for acute promyelocytic leukaemia with one study showing a 96% cure rate *(43)*

Vitamin A is found in two primary forms:

- Active vitamin A (i.e. retinol), which is derived from animal foods, such as liver and fish oils (especially cod) eggs and dairy

- Beta-carotene (a precursor of vitamin A), comes in a form that the body converts to retinol by normal metabolic processes as required. Beta-carotene is found in plant-based foods (see beta-carotene p.124)

## SAFETY ISSUES

While vitamins in general are much safer than drugs and rarely cause toxicity (even at very high levels), Vitamin A is the exception to the rule. High doses of supplemental vitamin A can be toxic to the body especially if a person has a compromised or diseased liver. Unless you are being medically supervised, if you do decide to use vitamin A supplements it is best to take low doses (800 micrograms) and top up with mixed carotenoids, allowing your body to make more vitamin A as the need arises. As an added safety, if you increase your intake of vitamin E, you'll be able to avoid any potential toxicity from high doses of vitamin A, since it is the lipid peroxide products from vitamin A utilisation that can cause damage to the liver. Vitamin E prevents lipid peroxidation.

# MINERALS WITH ANTI-CANCER PROPERTIES:

## SELENIUM

Selenium is a powerful mineral with anti-cancer properties. Needed only in very small amounts, it plays a crucial role in your cells' defences against cancer. It is a central part of the antioxidant enzyme glutathione peroxidise that eliminates free radicals, the unstable molecules that can damage your cells and ultimately lead to cancer. It also plays a role in re-activating spent antioxidants such as Vitamin E, which can then better perform their own anti-cancer functions.

Many studies over the last few decades have shown that selenium is a potent protective nutrient for some forms of cancer. As early as 1996 selenium supplementation was shown to lower overall cancer rates, with specific reductions in lung, colorectal and prostate cancers.[44]

Many large scale epidemiological studies have shown that populations with low selenium levels have a significantly increased risk of developing many different types of cancer. These studies show that having an adequate amount of dietary selenium can have preventative effects on most cancers. [45]

Detailed studies have shown that selenium acts through numerous ways to prevent cancers from developing. Scientists know of at least twelve distinct mechanisms by which selenium attacks cancer on many different fronts, and at many different stages. *(46)*

**They are:**

1. Regulation of lipoxygenase enzymes which produce inflammatory molecules that stimulate cancer growth
2. Reduction of oxidative stress that causes free radical damage
3. Protection of seleno-proteins, which recycle antioxidants
4. Detoxification of the body from cancer causing heavy metals
5. Induction of protective "phase 2" liver enzymes that neutralize many carcinogenic toxins
6. Inhibition of DNA alterations (genetic damage) which initiate cancerous changes in cells
7. Inactivation of molecular transcription factors required by cancer cells to support their growth and development
8. Shutting down of the essential cell replication cycle needed by cancer cells to produce their explosive growth
9. Induction of apoptosis, the programmed cell death, which is missing in cancer cells, allowing them to continue to reproduce indefinitely and potentially live forever
10. Enhanced immune system activity to detect and destroy incipient cancer cells
11. Down-regulation of sex hormone receptors used by certain cancers to sustain their growth
12. Limiting effects on tumour invasion and metastasis

Selenium occurs in multiple forms in nature, three of which are especially important in preventing cancer, they are:

- Sodium selenite
- L-selenomethionine

-   Selenium-methyl-selenocysteine

Each of these three forms of selenium confer a unique spectrum of cancer-preventative effects. So, only by combining all three forms can you be sure of optimizing your cancer risk reduction. In that way you'll be taking advantage of all of the twelve known mechanisms by which selenium compounds prevent and reverse cancer.

Daily dietary anti-cancer dose is 200 mcg

Brazil nuts, wheat germ, seafood, eggs, garlic, onions, brewers yeast, and chicken breast are the best sources of selenium.


# ZINC

Zinc is a multi-talented mineral found in all the body tissues and is imperative for healthy cell division and growth. It strengthens your immunity and even contributes to the production of proteins, including your DNA. It also helps in wound healing. It is a central component of the powerful antioxidant enzyme SOD (superoxide dismutase), which breaks down the free radical superoxide to form hydrogen peroxide ($H_2O_2$). $H_2O_2$ is deadly to cancer cells but not to normal cells (see Vit C for more info on $H_2O_2$). Zinc is also one of the key minerals for preventing cancer and stopping its spread.

Like selenium, zinc supports many aspects of the immune system and its deficiency can make us more vulnerable to cancer. A deficiency of zinc can lead to depressed activity of natural killer (NK) cells and other white blood cells.[47] Zinc deficiency and cancer are both common in the elderly. In one study researchers from the school of Medicine at the University of Michigan gave elderly people a daily zinc supplement over a one year period. They found that levels of pro-inflammatory markers and cancer promoting tumour necrosis factor (TNF) were significantly lower in the zinc-supplemental group than in the placebo group. Also these elderly individuals suffered fewer infections than the placebo group. [48]

Another American study speaks of how zinc can aid cancer treatment. The mineral reduces angiogenesis (the formation of new blood vessels that feed tumours) and induces cancer cell death (apoptosis).*(49)*

Researchers at the Rutgers Cancer Institute of New Jersey and Princeton University's prestigious Institute for Advance Studies have figured out one method by which zinc can shrink cancerous tumours. *(50)*

Here's how: Most solid-tumour cancers such as breast, prostate and ovarian develop because of a protein called P53. Known as the "guardian of the genome" (ie.DNA)*(51)* P53 controls the natural, programmed cell death called apoptosis. If P53 detects stress within a cell, it makes a call to either fix the cell or if the damage is significant, it triggers cell death.

But when cancer is present the gene that makes P53 is mutated or disabled. The mutated form of the P53 gene produces a damaged P53 protein that is no longer capable of signalling cell repair, nor can it intervene and trigger a cancer cell's death. The protein effectively unfolds, which makes it stop working.

What the researchers discovered, was that raising the amount of zinc in a cell, causes the P53 protein to fold right back up and function normally. From there, the recovered P53 protein can recognise the damage done to the cell by cancer, and prompt apoptosis.

More recently researchers have discovered another mechanism by which zinc attacks only cancer cells, but leaves healthy ones. The new research has tested the mineral on oesophageal cancer cells, although the researchers at the University of Texas led by Zui Pan, an associate professor of nursing, and a noted oesophageal cancer researcher, believes it would work just as well on other cancers.

The researchers discovered that cancer cells emit overactive calcium signals, and this attracts zinc which inhibits the cancer cell's growth. The researchers believe that calcium and zinc are somehow linked and "talk" to each other and this conversation inhibits cancer cell growth.

Without sufficient levels of zinc in the body this "crosstalk" and blocking process cannot happen effectively. "An insufficient amount of zinc can therefore lead to the development of cancer and other diseases" Pan said. Taking zinc supplements is an important part of the daily regime, the researchers say, as is eating foods that are rich in zinc such as spinach, beef, seafood like shellfish and oysters, eggs, pumpkin seeds, sunflower seeds and sesame seeds. *(52)*

# MAGNESIUM

Magnesium is a macro-mineral (meaning you need lots of it) that plays a role in over 300 different enzyme reactions in the body including igniting the "spark of life" to metabolic functions involving the creation of energy and its transport (ie. ATP- the body's energy currency). Every single cell in the human body demands adequate magnesium to function or it will perish. Strong bones and teeth, balanced hormones, a healthy nervous and cardiovascular system, well-functioning detoxification pathways, and much more depend upon cellular magnesium sufficiency. Magnesium also has a central role in regulating DNA synthesis and the cell cycle.

Without enough magnesium, the cell's sodium-potassium pump system will malfunction, allowing an intercellular buildup of sodium and calcium ions, turning the cells acidic and with lower oxygen. Indeed several studies have suggested that low magnesium will negatively affect the cell wall permeability, and this in itself can initiate cancer. *(53)*

Research into the effects of magnesium on cancer has been ongoing since the 1960s using animal studies which show that magnesium-deficient rats develop tumours of the thymus; an organ of the immune system needed to fight infections. *(54)* In animals, magnesium deficiency can spontaneously generate bone tumours and lymphomas. *(55)*

A systematic review published in the year 2011 by the International Society for the development of Research on Magnesium found that magnesium deficiency can lead to the initiation and proliferation of cancer, and that by optimising magnesium intake might prevent cancer or help in its treatment. *(56)*

A meta-analysis study published in September 2012 in the American Journal of Clinical Nutrition showed that higher intakes of magnesium correlated with a lower risk of colorectal cancer. (57)Results from the study indicated that for every 100mg increase in magnesium intake was associated with 12% lower risk of developing colorectal cancer.

A study published in 2000 found that almost half of cancer patients admitted to the intensive care unit had low magnesium levels. (58) Magnesium deficiency may have contributed to their disease but it may also have resulted from their cancer treatment. For example, cisplatin, a chemotherapy drug used to treat all types of cancer, can cause a number of serious side effects, including magnesium deficiency, in most cancer patients. The results of a 2008 study indicates that magnesium supplementation can prevent most of these side effects and decrease the severity of cisplatin-induced kidney damage without interfering with the anticancer effect of the drug. (59)

Other platinum-based drugs such as carboplatin, oxaliplatin, pyriplatin and phenanthriplatin, which are given to approximately half of all patients undergoing chemotherapy, have been shown in multiple studies to deplete magnesium levels in these patients. (60)

Symptoms of magnesium deficiency may include fatigue, muscle cramps, insomnia, irritability, weakness, depression, poor appetite, abnormal heart rate, headaches and nerve twitches.

Research has also shown that supplementing magnesium during platinum-based chemotherapy significantly reduces the degree of low magnesium levels. (61) It is recommended that everyone on this type of chemotherapy take 400mg daily of supplemental magnesium.

The best food sources of magnesium are organic green leafy vegetables (magnesium is found at the centre of every chlorophyll molecule: the green pigment in plants vital for the creation of energy from sunlight); nuts and seeds, such as almonds, sunflower, sesame and pumpkin seeds, kelp and other sea vegetables and avocados. Utilising bone broths on a daily basis will provide another excellent source of minerals, including magnesium, in a highly assimilable form.

Oral magnesium supplements are available in organic salt chelates, such as magnesium bisglycinate and magnesium citrate. These are very well absorbed, especially in powder forms to which you add water and can tailor your dosage. Another potential way to get more magnesium in your body is via the pleasant method of soaking in a bath of magnesium sulfate, otherwise known as Epsom salts. A couple of cups of Epsom salts added to a hot bath will induce sweating and detoxification, and after the water cools a bit the body will then absorb the magnesium sulphate.

Yet, another method to increase your magnesium levels is via the regular practice of Floatation Therapy wherein you lie suspended in a highly concentrated epsom salt solution, so dense that you float effortlessly. The solution is heated to 35 degrees celsius to match your body's skin temperature for maximum comfort. Apart from raising your magnesium levels, Floatation offers many other health benefits such as:

- Deep physical and mental relaxation
- Lowering of stress hormones
- Reduction of pain and inflammation
- Help in detoxification of the body
- Improvement of mental faculties
- Release of endorphins (the body's feel good hormone)
- Improvement in sleep patterns

To find out more about floatation therapy visit my website at www.naturaltherapy.ie/floatation-therapy/

# IODINE

Iodine is an essential mineral that most people are deficient in, and this deficiency can lead to cancers of the breast, prostate, ovaries, uterus, stomach and pancreas. Iodine's role in thyroid function is well known. It is part of the structure of the thyroid hormones T3 and T4 which regulate the body's energy usage (basal metabolism) along with many other important functions.

Iodine's protective role as an anti-cancer nutrient is just beginning to be widely appreciated in research circles. It is known to have antiseptic, antioxidant and anti-inflammatory properties, which may help in the treatment of cancer. It has also been shown to play a role in cell-differentiation and can induce apoptosis (cancer cell death).*(62)*

Epidemiological evidence points to iodine deficiency as a potential risk factor for cancer development. The evidence is strongest for breast and stomach cancer (both organs have a high number of iodine receptor sites) but emerging data indicate that iodine deficiency may also be a contributing factor in prostate, uterine, ovarian, thyroid and perhaps many other cancer types.*(62)*

Iodine can modify the effects of oestrogen on breast tissue, thus reducing fibrocystic breast disease, which doubles the risk for developing breast cancer.*(63)*

Japanese women (who eat lots of seaweed which is high in iodine) have the lowest incidence of breast cancer in the world. Iceland; another high iodine intake country also has low breast cancer rates.

Dr. David Brownstein, an expert on iodine and author of the book, "Iodine: Why You Need It, Why You Can't Live Without It" clearly explains what we would expect to find in iodine deficient individuals. *(64)*

He states that when iodine is deficient, nodules form in key organs leading to precancerous conditions and then eventually to full-blown cancer. He then goes on to explain that: *"Iodine's main job is to maintain a normal architecture of those tissues. With iodine deficiency the first thing that happens is you get cystic formation in the breasts, the ovaries, uterus, thyroid, prostate and, let's throw the pancreas in here as well, which is also increasing at epidemic rates - pancreatic cancer. Cysts start to form when iodine deficiency is there. If it goes on longer, they become nodular and hard. If it goes on longer, they become hyperplastic tissue which is the precursor to cancer. I say that's the iodine deficiency continuum."* Brownstein continues *"The good thing about iodine is iodine has apoptotic properties, meaning it can stop a cancer cell from just continually dividing until it kills somebody. Iodine can stop this continuum whenever it catches it and hopefully reverse it, but at least put the brakes on what is happening."*

Ultimately, the cause of all cancers is multifactorial, with benefit assumed in the elimination or reduction of modifiable risk factors. There is substantial evidence that iodine deficiency is a modifiable risk factor in cancer, especially of the breast and stomach and possibly many other organs.

The most effective anticarcinogenic form of iodine appears to be molecular iodine (I2). While it is generally considered that doses at 1100mcg as the safe upper limit, doses up to 4mg/50 kg body weight of I2 appear to be both safe and therapeutic for benign breast disease. (62) Doses above that range can produce side-effects including suppressed thyroid function.

Many of the iodine supplements on the market provide iodine in the form of potassium iodide. While this is safe in small doses (less than 1,100 mcg/day), the salts carry greater risk of interfering with thyroid function at higher doses. The ideal supplement would contain molecular iodine (I2) with very little iodide. The difficulty is that iodine I2 needs to be mixed with iodide in water to make it more soluble (ie. Lugol's solution). Given that whole food sources are generally safe, they are perhaps the best means of supplying iodine for the reduction in cancer risk. The best dietary sources are fish and sea vegetables, including seaweeds like kelp and wakame or kombu. Celtic sea salt contains a balance of a number of minerals including naturally occurring iodine.

## SUPPLEMENTS: HIGH QUALITY AND NATURAL - THE KEY

One of the most common mistakes people make is to buy the cheapest supplements on the market, thinking they're all the same. Most wouldn't even purchase toilet paper this way. As I've already outlined in this section, synthetic vitamins are not good for you. You may already have taken multivitamins and minerals for years figuring that they wouldn't hurt you. Unfortunately, research shows that taking these manufactured synthetic supplements is actually worse than not taking anything.

As I alluded to previously in the vitamin E segment of this chapter, two manufactured forms called DL-alpha-tocopherol and D-alpha-tocopherol acetate have no anticancer activity and are both absorbed poorly in the body. And in high doses they interfere with carotenoid absorption. Yet these are the most common (and cheap) forms sold to the public and used in human clinical trials, even though they are known to be toxic for human consumption.

On the other hand, a number of studies have demonstrated that natural forms of vitamin E (containing tocopherols and tocotrienols) have excellent anticancer effects, are well absorbed, boost immunity, reduce inflammation and are much more powerful as antioxidants.

The same can be said for beta-carotene. Synthetic beta-carotene is not only less active, but it can inhibit the activity of other vital anticancer nutrients. This synthetic form was used in a number of studies with claims that it increased the cancer rate amongst smokers, and there were more heart attacks and strokes in those who took the supplement (65)

However, a number of experiments using natural forms of beta-carotene (which naturally contains over a dozen forms) uncovered profound cancer inhibiting properties. Like synthetic vitamin E, synthetic beta-carotene obstructs the more active forms of the carotenoids such as alpha-carotene and lutein.

When buying a beta-carotene supplement select the natural form, which contains mixed carotenoids. It is usually extracted from an algae called Dunaliella salina.

Like I already said; when purchasing supplements; don't go cheap. Invest in high-end quality supplements based mostly on food concentrates. Nutrients derived from real foods are far healthier than man-made synthetic nutrients. It's important to know that not all natural supplements are created equal. Cheaper retail products made for the mass market may have ingredients whose quality and strength have been compromised. For instance, the manufacturing process may be speeded up, which can destroy some ingredients through excessive heat and compaction.

Also, low-cost products often contain reactive fillers and binders, which further reduce the expense of manufacturing. Reactive fillers commonly used to reduce expenses and bulk-up the product include talcum powder, shellac, hydrogenated oils, gluten, yeast and lactose. Unfortunately, these fillers reduce both the biological activity and clinical effectiveness of the nutrients.

Additionally, how the nutrient is bound will also make a difference for ease of absorption and utilization. For example, iron sulphate is a commonly used form of iron that irritates the intestines and may cause constipation. The source of the problem here is not the iron but the sulfate carrier. Other forms of iron such as iron glycinate are less likely to cause constipation. A rule of thumb, when taking minerals, is to take them as either: citrates, fumarates, gluconates, amino acid chelates or picolinates.

To identify if a nutrient is synthetic, check on the label to see if a source is given. If it isn't, assume the product is synthetic. Terms that can identify a vitamin as synthetic include: hydrochloride, chloride, acetate, bitartrate, nitrate and succinate. In the naturally occurring forms of vitamins, for example: Vitamin C complex, the ascorbic acid portion comprises only about 5% of the whole complex. Similarly, alpha-tocopherol only comprises a small percentage of vitamin E complex.

In conclusion, don't be hoodwinked into believing that large quantities of dead synthetic chemicals are more nutritionally potent than smaller amounts of high-quality natural living compounds. Relatively small amounts of whole-food natural nutrients with all of their naturally-occurring synergists are far more potent than high doses of synthetic imitation vitamins and metallic-based minerals. It is a natural law that you can't repair and rebuild a living body with dead synthetic chemicals. It simply isn't possible.

---
**CHAPTER 7**
---

# Beating Cancer with herbs

*"Behold, I have given you every green plant, and it shall be food
for you."* (Genesis 1:29)

**H**erbs have been used to treat all manner of ailments, including cancer, for thousands of years. Throughout history, various cultures have handed down their accumulated knowledge of the medicinal use of herbs to successive generations. This vast body of information serves as a basis for much of traditional medicine today.

Nowadays, this traditional use is also backed up by an enormous body of scientific information and research in the field of herbal medicine. Indeed many modern pharmaceuticals have been modelled on, or derived from chemicals found in plants. Some examples include the heart medication "digoxin" derived from foxglove (digitalis purpurea) and the analgesic "morphine", derived from the opium poppy (Papaver somniafera).

In the case of cancer, many chemotherapy drugs used to fight cancer are plant-derived agents. Some examples include:

- The chemotherapy drugs vincristine, vinblastine and vindesine, which are alkaloids derived from the Madagascar periwinkle plant.

- Taxanes (paclitaxel and docetaxel) are derived from the bark of the pacific yew tree, and are first choice chemotherapy drugs for treating breast, ovary, prostate, lung and other metastatic cancers
- The anticancer drug "podophyllotoxin" is derived from the roots of the may-apple (Podophyllum peltatum) and the Himalyan may-apple (Podophyllum hexandrum)
- The 'camptothecin' chemo-drugs come from a derivative of the Chinese happy tree

A great deal of pharmaceutical research is now focused on analysing the active ingredients of herbs to determine how and why they work. These ingredients are then isolated and/or synthetically replicated to produce potent chemotherapy drugs. The problem with this reductionist approach to making medicines is that these lab-produced anticancer compounds are very toxic to healthy cells in the body when used in isolation. By contrast, herbalists don't extract plant compounds in the way the drug industry does. They believe that herbal medicine works best when given in its whole unadulterated natural state. Because medical scientists tend to only look at the plants active compounds and isolate them, they tend to overlook and disregard all the other ingredients in the plant, which act to produce a modified and more balanced pharmacological response without the toxic side-effects that isolated active ingredients produce.

So far the pharmacological research done on known anticancer herbs has elucidated the various mechanisms by which they fight cancer malignancy. Anticancer herbs work by:

- Inhibiting cancer activating enzymes
- Promoting production of protective enzymes
- Stimulating DNA repair mechanisms
- Inducing antioxidant effects
- Modulating the activity of specific hormones that promote cancer growth
- Enhancing the activity of immune cells
- Enhancing detoxification functions of the body

- Reducing the toxic side effects of chemotherapy and radiotherapy

There are literally thousands of herbal remedies that have anti-cancer effects. The following list offers some of the better studied herbals. The studies listed below show that all herbs work in a different manner; and when combined, various herbal formulations have been specifically designed to attack cancerous tumours without harming normal cells of the body. This, of course, is the most desirable outcome when treating cancer.

# ASTRAGALUS (Astragaglus membranaceus)

Astragalus is a plant native to China and surrounding countries including Korea and Mongolia. It grows to approximately 1m in height over a four-year period whereupon the root being the medicinal part of the plant is harvested.

This root has been used for many hundreds of years both in Traditional Chinese Medicine (TCM) as a tonic for building both vitality and blood. It is widely regarded as an excellent "adaptogen" and immunostimulant herb. An adaptogen is a term given to herbs that have the ability to positively influence a wide range of biochemical processes in the body, in order to return body functions to their normal homeostatic (balanced) levels.

## Therapeutic uses of Astragalus

- The key notes for its use are chronic debility and immune depression
- Treatment of chronic infections and impaired immunity
- General debility and fatigue
- Excessive sweating
- Ischaemic heart disease
- Tonic for elderly patients

- Conditions/treatments resulting in immune suppression such as surgery, chemotherapy and radiotherapy

## Astragalus: Therapeutic Benefits for Cancer Patients

In numerous clinical studies, Astragalus has been shown to effect positive changes for people suffering from health conditions ranging from the common cold to cancer. For example, a clinical study involving 1000 people showed protection by astragalus against the common cold. [1] The subjects received astragalus either orally or as a nasal spray. A prophylactic effect for the common cold was observed as evidenced by decreased incidence and shortened duration of infection. The herb appeared to stimulate the production of an immune-boosting compound called "Interferon" that helped to deactivate the virus responsible for causing the common cold. Interferon is an important modulator of immune function and is also effective in preventing cell mutation and cancer development.

In Chinese studies, astragalus has been shown 'in vitro' (taking place in a test tube or petri dish) to promote interferon production. [2] Also, oral doses (ie. in vivo) of astragalus given to humans increased levels of all antibodies marketly.

In relation to cancer, a variety of human studies has shown astragalus to stimulate various parameters of the immune system; demonstrate anti-tumour activity, and inhibit the spreading of cancer to other areas of the body. [3]

In the USA researchers have looked at astragalus as a possible treatment for people whose immune systems have been damaged by chemotherapy and radiotherapy. These studies reveal that astragalus supplements seem to help these people recover faster and live longer. In one study, researchers from the University of Texas reported that cancer patients undergoing radiotherapy have twice the survival rate if they take astragalus compared to those receiving placebos.

This ability of astragalus to prolong life in cancer patients may be partly due to its ability to reduce the toxic side effects of conventional treatments. For instance, astragalus is known to improve liver function (often impaired in cancer patients). In one study conducted at the Peking Cancer Institute, researchers observed a much higher survival rate among terminal stage liver cancer patients when they received astragalus supplements along with their radiation treatment compared to those treated with radiation alone.*(4)*

In Chinese hospitals astragalus is routinely given to cancer patients to speed up recovery from the toxic side effects of radiation and chemotherapy. In one chinese study, patients with lung cancer who received a combination treatment of chemotherapy, radiotherapy, immunotherapy, and a herbal mixture consisting of astragalus and panax ginseng had improved survival rates with some patients living an extra 3 to 17 years. *(5)*

In a comparative Chinese study, an infusion of astragalus and ginseng in combination with chemotherapy reduced the toxic effects of the chemotherapy, increased body weight and increased cellular immune function compared to chemotherapy alone in 176 patients with colon cancer.*(6)*

In light of the above studies and the mountains of ongoing research on the health benefits of astragalus, could we consider it to be the herb that prevents and also cures cancer? To answer that question we need to consider the properties of an effective anticancer remedy. Medical herbalists agree that a herb needs to possess two very important therapeutic requirements when treating cancer:

    1.   Immuno - modulating action

    2.   Adaptogenic action

Astragalus has demonstrated its ability to do both jobs synergistically, ie; in a more cooperative fashion. The thing is cancer cells have the ability to hide from the immune system, so it is not enough to just simulate immune function in order to beat cancer. We have to de-cloak the cancer cells so they appear on the immune system's radar screens.

Not only does astragalus increase white blood cell counts along with other immune modulators, including antibody levels, its adaptogenic properties helps the immune system differentiate between healthy cells and cancer cells, thereby boosting the body's total cancer fighting system. Astragalus, no doubt is a useful herb to add to your arsenal of remedies in the fight against cancer, but to consider it in isolation as a cure for cancer would be stretching the imagination somewhat....

## Pharmacodynamics - How Astragalus works

Astragalus works by stimulating several factors of the immune system. Its poly-saccharides (Active constituents) show considerable immune-enhancing activity in vitro (test tube). Laboratory results show that these polysaccharides:

- Increase the immune-mediated anti-tumour activity of interleukin-2 compounds
- Improves the response of lymphocytes (a type of white blood cell) in both normal and cancer patients alike.
- Enhances natural killer (NK) cell activity and potentiates activity of monocytes (two types of white blood cells) [7]

## Dosage and Administration

Traditionally Astragalus would be taken as the powdered dried root in the dosage range 10 to 30grams per day. In liquid form the adult dosage is 4 to 8ml per day of the 1:2 fluid extract.

## BAICAL SCULLCAP (Scuttellaria biacalensis)

For more than 2000 years Baical scullcap, a member of the mint family, also known as Chinese scullcap (Huang gin in Chinese) has remained one of the most highly regarded herbs in traditional Chinese medicine. It is a perennial plant, native to China and Russia, which grows to the height of 1 metre. Its purple flowers are characterized by a specific shape, which resembles a skull, hence its common name. Its roots are thick and branchy and are the part of the plant that's used for medicinal purposes. The roots are harvested after four years of growth as that's when it has the highest amount of beneficial agents.

Its root is almost skinless and is a rich source of over 35 flavonoids, giving it a yellow colour, hence its traditional name of golden root or 'huang gin' the Chinese word for yellow gold. The major constituents of baical scullcap are Wogonin, Baicalein and Baicalin. [8]

All researchers of this plant agree that these flavonoids are the main chemicals which display beneficial effects in the human body. One of these flavonoids in particular is 'baicalein', which is being studied for its anti-cancer, anti-inflammatory, antiviral, antibacterial and antiallergy effects. Research done on cells cultured in the lab (in vitro) has shown that these flavonoids can kill human cancers while leaving healthy cells untouched. This is no doubt partly down to scullcap's strong antioxidant activity, which has been shown to protect the cells DNA from free radical damage. In vitro evidence also indicates the flavonoid baicalein can stimulate DNA repair enzymes. [9]

Another anti-cancer mechanism of action that is attracting a great deal of attention from the scientific community is baicalein's ability to halt the replication of various human cancer cell lines via the inhibition of the 12 lipooxygenase enzyme system. [10] Studies show that by blocking this particular enzyme, cancer cells cannot replicate and are also forced into a apoptosis (programmed cell death). In addition, the spread of cancer cells to other tissues (metastasis) is severely curtailed.

Another mechanism of action by which baicalein inhibits the replication of cancer cells is by directly or indirectly inhibiting specific enzymes (ie. protein tyrosine kinase and protein Kinase C) required for cellular division and proliferation of cancer cells. [17]

A study carried out by researchers from Mount Sinai School of Medicine at New York University found that biacal scullcap strongly inhibits cell growth in all cancer cell lines tested. They believe one mechanism of action is baicalein's ability to suppress the production of prostaglandin - two compounds which fuel tumour growth. They also found that prostate and breast cancer cells were more sensitive to the treatment than other cell types. [12]

Another interesting study [12] found that baicalein inhibits the 5 alpha-reductase enzyme which is responsible for converting testosterone to dihydrotestosterono (DHT). DHT is strongly associated with the development of prostate enlargement and prostate cancer, two health problems that many elderly men suffer from. I always include this miracle herb in formulas when men present with these conditions.

## Human Studies

Baical scullcap has not been studied in clinical trials as a single agent, but has been studied in combination with other herbal formulations. [13] I personally think this is the best way to take herbs, as the effect is to increase the magnification of all the active compounds through synergism.

The term synergism may be defined as the harmonious action of two or more active constituents that produce an effect, which neither could produce alone, or an effect, which is greater than the total effects of each constituent operating by itself.

In a prospective study performed by researchers from the University of California in conjunction with Memorial Sloan-Kettering Cancer Center in New York, an herbal mixture containing baicalein extract was given to men suffering from advanced prostate cancer, and which was unresponsive to chemotherapy drugs and other medical interventions. The herbal tonic was shown to significantly improve the men's condition. After a year on this tonic all patients with testosterone driven cancer had a decline of 80% or more in their prostate-specific antigen (PSA) levels. Of two patients with metastasis (cancer spread) to the bone, one experienced a complete disappearance of cancerous bone lesions and the other showed good improvement. Another patient's bladder tumour completely disappeared. [14] Other studies involving men with prostate cancer who were taking this particular herbal formula have demonstrated similar results.

## Dosage:

The usual doses for therapeutic purposes range from 2 to 6 grams/day of the dried root or 4 to 12 ml/day of the 1:2 fluid extract.

# BLOODROOT (Sanguinaria canadensis)

Bloodroot is a perennial wildflower that grows in woodlands in North America. Its healing power lies in its root system that comprise of a stout rhizome, which oozes with a bright red sap when cut, hence the name bloodroot. The root and rhizome are harvested in the autumn for medicinal use.

Bloodroot contains a variety of chemicals including one particularly beneficial plant alkaloid called sanguinarine. Sanguinarine has been shown to possess anti-microbial[15] tumour-cidal (cancer killing)[16, 17] anticancer and anti-inflammatory properties [18] which has given bloodroot its medicinal value as an antiseptic against various infections and as a chemo-therapautic agent in the fight against cancer.

# How does Sanguinarine in Bloodroot kill cancer cells?

Various researchers studying the mechanisms of sanguinarine have discovered that it works in a variety of ways to directly kill cancer cells as well as inhibit its growth. [19] One way that sanguinarine makes cancer cells vulnerable to destruction is its ability to inhibit the production of a protein called "survivin". [20] Cancer cells produce survivin to enhance their cellular division and also to protect themselves from undergoing the normal process of cell death (apoptosis). Without survivin as their protective sheath cancer cells soon become subject to the normal cycles of cell death.

As you probably know by now, new blood vessel formation within cancerous tumours is an essential physiological process for the tumour to grow. This process is called angiogenesis. Researchers have discovered a proangiogenic molecule within tumours called Vascular Endothelial Growth Factor (VEGF) that is a major driver of tumour angiogensis.[21] Sanguinarine is able to inhibit VEGF activity thereby stopping the new growth of blood vessels within tumours.[22, 23] By doing so, the tumour is effectively starved to death.

Sanguinarine can also directly kill cancer cells through a variety of molecular mechanisms. A 2013 study published in the European Journal of Pharmacology showed that sanguinarine causes cancer cell death through selective oxidative damage. *(24)* Another 2012 Korean study published in the Journal of Toxicology discovered that sanguinarine can stimulate apoptosis through the "activation of caspase cascade pathways", which are key executioners in apoptosis.*(25)*

## Dosage Precautions

Bloodroot is a potentially toxic herb, so self-medication should be avoided. Take internally only under the guidance of a healthcare professional knowledgeable in herbalism. When taken in excess, bloodroot can cause nausea and make you vomit. It can also cause burning in the stomach, abnormal heart rhythms and visual distortions. However, when used in the correct dosage and in combinations with other anticancer herbs, its efficacy as a cancer fighter is beyond question.

## CANCER BUSH (Sutherlandia frutescens)

Cancer bush is a shrub native to South Africa and along the coast of West Africa. It has been used for centuries in the traditional system of medicine of the native peoples and the European colonists. Its common name is derived from the belief that it cured cancer. It has powerful immune boosting properties and has been classified as an adaptogen.

> An Adaptogen is a herbal substance that helps the body to adapt to environmental and internal stress by changing body metabolism. Adaptogens generally work by strengthening the immune system, nervous system and / or glandular system.

## Traditional uses of Cancer Bush

Cancer bush has application in the treatment of all conditions that are associated with impaired immune function and general debility of the body. It strengthens the body's immune system and acts as a general tonic to accelerate the recovery process.

It has been used traditionally by the natives to treat a number of ailments including:

- Cancer (the reason for its local name as the 'cancer bush')
- Colds and flu
- Diabetes
- Arthritis
- Viral infections ( inc. hepatitis and HIV/Aids)
- Asthma and bronchitis
- Blood pressure
- Digestive disorders

Scientific research and clinical experience suggests that the key constituents in cancer bush exhibit the following properties:

- Immunomodulatory
- Anti-inflammatory
- Anti-viral
- Anti-bacterial
- Anti-fungal
- Anti-cancer
- Vaso-dilatory [26]

Here is a summary of research into Cancer Bush's health benefits as published in various journals:

A paper entitled "In vitro culture studies of Sutherlandia frutescens on human tumour cell lines", published in the Journal of Ethnopharmacology found that Cancer Bush inhibited the proliferation of several human tumour cell lines by as much as fifty percent. [27]

Another in vitro study in the same Journal of Ethnoparmacology found that Cancer Bush can kill cervical and ovarian cancer cells. [28] It should be noted that these studies only look at the effect of Cancer Bush on cancer cells growing in a laboratory and not its effect on cancer growing in the body.

Yet another in-vitro study in the same above journal showed that Cancer Bush extract inhibited the growth of breast cancer cells by inducing them to self-destruct (apoptosis). *(29)*

There are also case studies of Cancer Bush's ability to reduce fatigue in cancer patients. *(30)*

It is well-known that cancer ravishes the body with most cancer patients succumbing to the wasting syndrome of weight loss, rather than the actual tumour mass.Tests show that the use of cancer bush dramatically improves the appetite and wasted patients start to gain weight by as much as 1kg per week. Rest assured though: when taken by those who do not have an underlying condition, Cancer Bush does not cause weight gain. *(31)*

Importantly, while evidence indicates that Cancer Bush has an anti-cancer effect and stimulates the immune system, it should not be regarded as a miracle cure for cancer. Its real benefits are as a tonic that will assist the body to mobilize its own resources (the immune system) to cope with the illness.


## Dosage:

The therapeutic dose of Cancer Bush for general well-being is 300mg of the dried extract twice daily with meals. This can be taken long term. Cancer patients may need to take 600 mg 3 times a day long-term to benefit from its anti-cancer properties.


## CAT'S CLAW (Uncaria tomentosa)

Cat's claw also known as "Una de Gato" from where it originates in Spanish speaking Peru, is a thick woody vine, the bark of which has been used in traditional medicine for many centuries to help heal a vast assortment of ailments. The name Cat's claw derives from the unique shape of the hook-like thorns found on this vine, which resemble the claws of a cat.

## History

The priests of the Ashaninka Indian tribe in Central Peru considered Cat's claw to have great powers and health improving properties, and so used this herb to ward off all manner of disease. They drank a tea made by boiling the inner bark of the Cat's claw vine.

It was in the 1920's when a German naturalist called Dr. Arturo Brell who was working in the Peruvian rain forest, first heard about the wonderful healing powers of this vine. At the time he was suffering from a painful episode of rheumatoid arthritis, so he decided to drink Cat's claw tea and before long he was cured of his arthritis. The bark worked because of its natural anti-inflammatory effect. Around the same time Dr. Brells friend Luis Schular was diagnosed with end stage lung cancer, and so hearing about Brell's success he decided to try the Cat's claw remedy. Schular drank this tea three times daily for one year and not only did his cancer regress during that time; it completely disappeared for good by the end of that year!

## Healing Claims

Cat's claw has been traditionally used as an anti-inflammatory, antiviral, immunostimulant, contraceptive and cancer remedy. *(32)* Proponents claim that it has helped people to overcome numerous conditions from arthritis, allergies and asthma, to viral infections, menstrual irregularities and even cancer. This wide array of therapeutic uses for Cat's claw is attributed to its many properties which are:

- Adaptogen
- Immune stimulant
- Antiviral
- Antimicrobial
- Antioxidant
- Anti-tumour

## Cancer fighting properties of Cat's claw

The therapeutic effect of Cat's claw for treating a variety of cancers including breast cancer, lung cancer, brain cancer, and leukaemia is well-known in South America and well studied by Brazilian researchers. It has several groups of plant chemicals that account for its action, the most studied group being oxidole alkaloids, which have been documented to have immunostimulant and anticancer properties. (33, 34, 35)

According to several early studies, Cat's claw treatment has been shown to lead to the remission of brain tumours and other types of cancers. (36) More recent studies and research on Cat's claw validate those earlier studies. A 2013 clinical study involving breast cancer patients demonstrated that the bark of Cat's claw prevented the growth of breast tumours due to modulation of oxidative stress among constituents with antioxidant properties.(37) A 2001 in vitro (test tube) study demonstrated that Cat's claw directly inhibited the growth of human breast cancer cell line by 90% by having anti-mutagenic and anti-metastic effects on the cancer cells. (38)

In a small Brazilian study of 40 breast cancer patients published in the journal Evidence-based Complementory and Alternative Medicine, Cat's claw reduced the adverse effects due to chemotherapy. Lab results at the end of the trial showed that the women in the herbal treatment group experienced less damage to the white blood cell count (ie. better immunity). There was also evidence that the Cat's claw was also able to repair cellular DNA damage caused by the chemotherapy drugs. (39)

A 1998 lab study by Swedish researchers reported on Cat's claw ability to inhibit the growth of lymphoma and leukaemia cell lines. A subsequent in vitro study published in the British Journal of Haematology also demonstrated its ability to fight against leukemia. The oxindole alkaloids of Cat's claw were able to inhibit the growth of human leukaemia cells and also induce cells to undergo apoptosis (commit suicide). (40)

More recently a 2015 study also found that Cat's claw is beneficial to terminal cancer patients by improving their quality of life and reducing side effects of chemotherapy and radiation such as nausea, secondary infections and fatigue. *(41)*

**Dosage:**

Scientific studies have shown that therapeutic effects against cancer tumours are observed when a 100mg dose of a dry extract of Cat's claw are taken three times daily.

# GINKGO BILOBA

The Ginkgo biloba tree is one of the oldest living species on earth with its lineage dating back 200 million years. A single tree can live as long as 1000 years and grow to a height of 35 metres. In China and Japan the tree has been cultivated in temple gardens for many centuries. It was introduced to Europe from the Far East around 1730 and is now widely cultivated in many countries around the world. *(42)*

Its seeds and leaves contain a wide assortment of chemical compounds which have been indispensable in traditional Chinese medicine for 5000 years, recommended for coughs, poor circulation, asthma, cardiovascular disorders, memory loss, low immunity and acute or sudden allergic inflammation.

Since its introduction into Europe, a great deal of attention has been focused on the therapeutic effects of Ginkgo leaves, with over 1,000 scientific studies being published in the last 50 years demonstrating its medicinal value. Most of these studies have been carried out on standardized extracts of the leaf and the current clinical use of ginkgo is based on this research and not so much on traditional use.

## How Ginkgo Biloba fights cancer

There is now a large and growing body of evidence to show that Ginkgo has powerful anti-cancer properties. According to Memorial Sloan Kettering Cancer Centre, Ginkgo extracts exhibit anti-infective, chemopreventative, anti-cancer and cytotoxic (poison cancer cells) effects in laboratory studies. *(43)*

The primary mechanisms of action through which these properties work are:

1. Powerful anti-oxidant effects
2. Strong anti-inflammatory activity
3. Promotes cancer cell apoptosis (cell suicide)
4. Inhibits angiogensis (new blood vessel formation)
5. Stabilizes damaged DNA

Ginkgo's anti-cancer activity is attributed to two major constituent groups called flavonoids and ginkgolides. The flavonoids are potent antioxidants that provide cellular protection against the damaging effects of harmful free radicals. In this way, these potent antioxidants, by preventing damage to the cells DNA are believed to help reduce the risk of cancer.

The ginkgolides also have powerful antioxidant activity in their own right and they have also been shown to improve blood flow by dilating blood vessels and reducing the stickiness of the platelets. Ginkgolide B, in particular apparently works by interfering with a chemical in the body known as PAF (platelet activating factor). PAF is a phospholipid compound released from Ig E antibody - activated basophils (a type of white blood cell) that causes the release of histamine (pro-inflammatory compound) from platelets causing them to clump together and become sticky. Cancer cells can then easily stick to these clumps and be carried around circulation (ie. metastize). PAF levels tend to be markedly higher in cancer patients compared to healthy people. It is believed that PAF is a stimulator of malignant tumour growth by way of stimulating inflammation and inducing angiogensis (the development of new blood vessels in tumours). *(44)* By suppressing PAF activity, Ginkgo helps to reduce inflammation and allergic reactions.

Ginkgo is also an excellent vasodilator meaning it expands the tiny blood vessels that nourish the body's tissues thus bringing oxygen and nutrients to the cells. In doing so, tissues and organs are better able to detoxify, resulting in an improved pH balance; remember cancer thrives in an acid environment.

Clinical trials with standardized Ginkgo leaf extract have confirmed its place in the clinical treatment of cancer. In a study published in 2003, in World Journal of Gastroenterol, researchers found that Ginkgo biloba reduced stomach tumours by a dramatic 73.4% in thirty patients with gastric cancer. *(45)*

In another study published in 2005 in "Oral Oncology", researchers found that Ginkgo leaf extracts induced apoptosis (cell suicide) in oral cancer cells by activating a compound called caspase-3. The researchers concluded that Ginkgo extract may be a possible anticancer agent against oral cavity cancer. *(46)*

In yet another study reported on, Drs. Bin Ye and Daniel Cramer studied a population of women that included 600 ovarian cancer cases and 640 healthy matched controls. Of the women who took Ginkgo supplements for a minimum of six months or longer, they were shown to have a 60% lower risk of developing ovarian cancer. *(47)*

In one well-known 1995 study, published in "Radiation Research" Chernobyl accident recovery workers were given Ginkgo extract over a period of two months, which reduced their high levels of clastogenic factors to normal levels. Clastogenic factors are biomarkers of oxidative damage that appear in the blood of people who have been irradiated. After treatment was stopped the normal levels persisted for seven months. *(48)*

**In conclusion,** Ginkgo biloba has been extensively researched and shown to have definite anti-cancer properties and I would recommend you add it to your anti-cancer programme and supplement regime.

# GREEN TEA (Camellia sinensis)

Regularly drinking green tea is another key element of cancer prevention. Researchers have long known of the relationship between those who consume green tea on a regular basis and their lowered incidence of cancer. According to traditional Chinese medicine, green tea possesses stimulant, digestive, diuretic and anti-toxic properties.

Since the 1970s the health effects of green tea were the subject of a lot of scientific studies. The results of those investigations confirmed its traditional uses and highlighted other pharmacological properties such as: cholesterol lowering, inhibits platelet adhesion, immune boosting, liver protecting, protection from radiation and anti-cancer properties. In human studies, those who regularly consume green tea have about half the cancer incidence of non green tea drinkers. *(49)*

Tea, both green and black comes from the plant Camellia sinensis, an evergreen shrub in which the young leaves can be either:

- Lightly steamed to produce green tea;
- Air dried and fermented to produce black tea

The steaming process deactivates enzymes in the leaf that would otherwise convert the plants potent antioxidants (ie. polyphenols) to less beneficial compounds.

Green tea contains a large group of plant compounds called polyphenols that include the catechins, which are believed to be responsible for the reputed health benefits that have traditionally been attributed to green tea. *(50)*

Six catechins have been isolated and identified from green tea. Epigallo-catechin-3-gallate (EGCG) is the most powerful and abundant catechin in green tea and accounts for 50-75% of its total catechin content.

The catechins are powerful anti-oxidants and are considered many times stronger than vitamin C and E in defending the body against damaging free radicals. *(51)* In a 1997 study, researchers from the University of Kansas determined that EGCG is twice as powerful as resveratrol (an ingredient found in the skin of red grapes) which itself is known to kill cancer cells.

EGCG is the most powerful green tea antioxidant and has been tested extensively over the past 20 years for cancer killing abilities. It has been shown to kill many different types of cancer cells in laboratory conditions.

- For instance: EGCG has substantial free radical scavenging capability, meaning this catechin can mop up damaging oxidative compounds that would otherwise cause damage to the DNA of cells. *(52)*

- The catechins in green tea can activate detoxification enzymes in the liver, such as glutathione S-transferase and quinone reductase; these enzymes inhibit tumour growth *(53)*
- Green tea catechins are capable of inhibiting tumour cell development and induce apoptosis (cancer cell destruction) in laboratory and animal studies. *(54)*
- Induction of new blood vessel growth, known as angiogensis, is required for tumour growth and metastasis. Studies show that the catechins and especially, EGCG prevents this growth of new blood vessels and cancerous tumours by as much as 70%.*(55)*
- The catechins in green tea can also protect cells from the damaging effects of ultra-violet radiation as well as protecting immune cells for a higher tumour-kill rate. *(56)*

## Clinical studies

For the most part, the evidence for EGCG and the other catechins anti-cancer activity comes mainly from laboratory and animal studies. Because of these promising results, many human clinical trials have been carried out to see if green tea consumption can indeed protect us from the risk of developing cancer. Some of the specific cancers where risk reduction has been clinically demonstrated include:

- Prostate cancer: In a large Japanese study, Japan being the country where studying consumption of green tea is easiest, it was shown that Japanese men who drank 5 or more cups of green tea per day had a 50% lower risk of developing prostate cancer. *(57)*

In a smaller double-blind, placebo controlled study comprising 60 men at high risk of developing prostate cancer; 30 of them received 200mg of green tea catechin supplements three times daily for one year, while the other group of 30 men received a placebo. After one year, only one man in the green tea catechin group developed prostate cancer compared to 9 men in the placebo group who developed prostate cancer. *(58)*

- Breast Cancer: A Japanese study done on women already diagnosed with breast cancer, whose disease was in its early stages and had not yet spread found that those who consumed at least three cups of green tea daily had 57% fewer relapses than women who drank one cup or less per day. *(59)*

A meta-analysis of multiple clinical studies also concluded that women who drank the most green tea had a substantially reduced risk of developing breast cancer compared to women who consumed black tea.*(60)*

- Bowel Cancer: A study of 69,710 chinese women aged 40 to 70 years found that green tea drinkers had a 57% lower risk of getting bowel cancer. *(61)*
- Bladder Cancer: A study of 882 women showed that those who regularly consumed green tea had a significantly reduced risk of getting bladder cancer. *(62)*

So the evidence is definitely in; while it may sound crazy, scientific research confirms that regularly drinking something as common as green tea can put you at a lesser risk of developing cancer. You don't even need to drink gallons to help your body kill cancer cells. Studies show that just two cups per day is enough to significantly increase the antioxidant catechin concentrations in your body. *(63)*

Of course it goes without saying that not all green teas are created equal. Matcha green tea is made from organic leaves grown in Japan, and is regarded as the gold standard of green teas. It is said that drinking one cup of matcha is equivalent to drinking at least ten cups of regular green tea. In fact a study conducted at the University of Colorado reported that matcha green tea has 137 times as much EGCG than regular green tea. *(64)*

# PAU D'ARCO - (Tabebuia Impetiginosa)

Much has been said of this herbal extract from the inner bark of the Tabebuia tree, found in South America rainforests. There are anedotal reports of widespread use to heal cancer with miraculous shrinkage and elimination of tumours. It is believed its anti-cancer activity is due to its main active ingredient, a substance called lapachol *(65, 66)*. In addition it contains many other active constituents making it effective as an anti-fungal, anti-viral, anti-bacterial and anti-parasitic remedy. These powerful ingredients contained in Pau d'arco have led consumers to use this herb for a wide variety of conditions, including candidiasis (yeast overgrowth), compromised immune systems, parasitic infections and cancer.

## Anti-tumour activity of Pau D'arco

Pau d'arco has been used for a long time in Latin America to treat cancer. As far back as 1962 the National Cancer Institute in America documented information on its use in Brazilian hospitals against cancer of the tongue, throat, esophagus, intestines, lung, head, prostate and leukaemia.

There was a small clinical trial in Brazil where nine patients were given pure lapachol in 250-mg capsules with meals. All nine patients showed shrinkage of tumours and reduction in pain. Three patients who had cancers of the mouth, the intestines and kidney had complete remission, and there were no adverse side effects reported during the trial. *(67)*

According to the American Cancer Society the constituent lapachol was found to fight against certain tumour cells in laboratory animals. In studies of mice injected with leukaemia cells, the life span of the mice receiving lapachol was 80% greater than that of the control group. *(68)*

The herbal extract also killed mice cancer cells both in culture and in the mice. The Pau d'arco extract also inhibited lung metastasis (spread of cancer to other organs) in mice following surgery to remove these cancer tumours. A 2005 study published in Oncology Reports found that lapachol has great potential as an application in fighting metastasis. *(69)*

Although there are only a few clinical studies (most done over thirty years ago) that verify the anti-cancer, anti-viral, anti-fungal, anti-bacterial and anti-parasitic activity of this South American herb, those who have experienced health changing benefits from its use, attest to its healing powers despite the lack of medical documentation.

Saying that, Pau d'arco should not be relied upon as a sole treatment for cancer. The therapeutic effects of its inner bark are likely to be mild and so drinking a tea made from this bark needs to be long-term. The good news is that by taking it this way holds far fewer toxic hazards that the regular consumption of coffee.

# PANAX GINSENG

Panax Ginseng is one of the oldest most widely used, and scientifically studied herb on this planet. For over 2,000 years Chinese doctors have prescribed ginseng for nearly every conceivable ailment. It has been used as a general tonic to improve the immune system, promote strength and vitality, improve appetite and better digestion, regulate glucose metabolism, enhance sexual performance, and to decrease stress. *(70)*

Panax ginseng is an ideal 'adaptogen'. An adaptogen is a substance, which can facilitate a non-specific increase in the resistance of an organism to noxious influences including physical, chemical, and biological stresses. *(71)* Panax ginseng is a plant species of which there are different varieties called:

- American ginseng (Panax quinquefolium)
- Japanese ginseng (Panax japonicum)
- Himalayan ginseng (Panax pseudoginseng)
- Chinese/Korean ginseng (Panax trifolium) *(72)*

Ginseng's therapeutic value comes from the 13 different triterpenoid saponins, collectively known as ginsenasides, which are found in its roots. It can be consumed as a tea, taken in capsule form or as a tincture.

## Scientific Evidence of Panax ginseng's Cancer-killing Properties

Chinese doctors have been using ginseng to treat cancer for over 2,000 years because of its unique adoptogenic qualities and ability to strengthen the immune system to fight rogue cancer cells. Fast forward to today where literally new studies are being published every day regarding its anti-inflammatory (inflammation being a major promoter of cancer growth) and antioxidant properties. New research is also demonstrating ginsengs ability to kill cancer cells, as well as inhibit cancers uncontrolled growth and ability to develop new blood vessels for nourishment.

According to a review study published in the Chinese Medicine Journal entitled "Ginseng's secret weapon for fighting cancer is revealed through its compound called ginsenosides", a team of researchers from the UK, China and Hong Kong reveal that compounds called ginsenosides are the plants secret weapon for fighting cancer. *(73)*

The studies demonstrate the beneficial effect of the ginsenosides against deviant molecular processes within cancer cells. The researchers identified four ways ginsenosides may shut down cancer cells:

1. **Inhibit cancer's uncontrolled growth**. Ginsenosides have been shown to halt the growth of tumours in the liver, lungs and prostate, as well as leukaemia cells.

2. **Cause cell death.** Ginseng has been shown to stimulate particular types of white blood cells called macrophages and NK cells (big eaters) to gobble up cancer cells and cell debris. In addition the ginsenosides cause apoptosis (normal self-destruction or programmed cell death) in a variety of different cancers.

3. **Stop cancer metastasis (invasive spreading).** Cancer cells can break away from their primary site and spread to other parts of

the body via the bloodstream or lymphatic system. From here, these wandering cells can form secondary tumours within the body. But researchers have observed that ginsengosides can stop cancer cells from spreading to secondary sites.

4. **Inhibit angiogenesis.** Angiogenesis is the term used for the development of new blood vessels and is the method by which cancer tumours nourish themselves. By inhibiting new blood vessel growth in tumours, cancer cells are less likely to grow. The report authors said that a number of studies have shown that certain metabolites of ginsenosides have been discovered to inhibit angiogenesis.

Panax ginseng can also bestow other therapeutic benefits on cancer patients via the following mechanisms:

- **Adaptogenic qualities:** The great diversity of pharmalogical properties attributed to ginseng makes it unsurpassed in the plant kingdom for its ability to act in a unique and fundamental way to rebalance the body's systems.
- **Liver Metabolism:** Ginseng stimulates DNA and protein synthesis in the liver *(74)* and helps protect the liver from chemically-induced damage. *(75)* Ginseng also activates immune cell scavengers in the liver called kupffer cells, which are responsible for house-cleaning in the body's most important detoxifying organ.
- **Blood sugar regulator:** Since cancer thrives on sugar, it stands to reason to keep blood sugar levels within normal limits in the cancer patient. Ginseng has been shown to significantly reduce fasting blood glucose levels in both diabetes and those fed on a high sugar diet.*(76)*

# Clinical Studies

37 cases of chemotherapy-induced immune damage were treated with ginseng. The treatment increased the white blood cell count to normal levels within two weeks in 82% of patients without any negative side

effects. *(77)*

Ginseng has been shown to improve brain function and immune function in 127 cases of elderly patients with cancer. *(78)*

Regular use of Ginseng can cut one's cancer risk in half according to a Korean retrospective study conducted on 1,987 pairs of individuals. This epidemiological study has shown that patients taking ginseng for one year had a 36% lower risk of cancer recurrence compared to patients not taking ginseng; and those who took ginseng for five years or more had a 69% lower cancer rate.*(79)*

Another epidemiologic study done in China with a cohort of 1,455 women with breast cancer showed improved survival and quality of life with regular ginseng use.*(80)*

Ginseng used in combination with chemotherapy drugs has been shown to act synergistically and increase the effectiveness of those drugs. In one study where patients took ginseng tablets for 30 days, they had little or no side effects from the chemo-drugs. The white blood cell count in these patients in the study increased by 65%.*(81)*

Based on well-established traditional use as well as modern clinical trials, panax ginseng is one of the most beneficial herbs to use in both prevention and treatment of cancer. Although there is no conclusive evidence of panax ginseng curing cancer as a stand-alone remedy (and I don't believe such a remedy exists, herbal or otherwise), it can be combined with other herbal medicines as well as other harmless natural treatments.

## Dosage and Dosage forms:

The adult dose is from 0.5 to 3.0 grams per day of the dried root, or 1 to 6ml per day of the 1:2 fluid extract. Since Panax ginseng has stimulatory properties, I recommend it be taken in the morning and early afternoon.

# AGLYCON SAPOGENIN (AGS)

The ginsenoside compounds in Panax ginseng consists of a sugar and a non-sugar component. The non-sugar component is called an Aglycon Sapogenin (AGS). There are many different kinds of AGS but the kind designated by the letter "R" have been shown to exhibit high-level anti-cancer activity. Researchers have used these AGS on deadly skin melanomas and observed these cancer cells die within 24 hours of contact.

Among the anti-cancer characteristics of Aglycon Sapogenin (AGS) are:

1. AGS stops cancer cell proliferation and induces cancer cell apoptosis (programmed cell death) through multiple mechanisms

2. AGS acts as chemosensitizers. Cancer cells are often genetically resistant or develop resistance to chemotherapy drugs during treatment. AGS can work with chemotherapy agents to enhance the efficacy of treatment and overcome the multi-drug resistance of cancer cells to chemotherapy.

3. AGS is a non-toxic, natural chemotherapy agent. AGS attacks only cancer cells with no harm to normal cells. AGS is even able to change cancer cells back into normal cells.

4. AGS interacts with the P450 enzyme system to reduce the production of carcinogens in our body and therefore may decrease the potential risk of getting cancer.

5. AGS is a potential cancer prevention agent. Prevention is the ultimate approach in the battle against cancer and AGS has been shown to protect you from developing malignant cancer cells in the first place.

The only down-side to AGS is its cost. In order to obtain one gram of the R-type AGS, hundreds of ginseng plants would be required. One company that produces a high quality AGS derived product is "Pegasus Pharmaceuticals Group" based in Canada. They produce AGS in both liquid and capsule form called Careseng SG2, it is made up of compounds derived from Panax ginseng which are structurally comparable to R-type AGS.

## SIBERIAN GINSENG (Eleutherococcus senticosus)

Siberian ginseng is not to be confused with Panax ginseng as it is from a different species altogether. It does however contain some ginseng-like compounds (triterpenoid saponins) that give it adaptogenic qualities).

While Siberian ginseng has no direct cancer killing effect, it has been shown to stimulate immunity in people with cancer *(82)*. It stimulates the anti-neoplastic (cancer fighting) activity of natural killer cells of the immune system, and may also help regenerate these same cells damaged by conventional treatments. When given to cancer patients, it minimises the side effects from chemotherapy, radiation and surgery, and improved healing and well being. Survival time in patients with terminal cancer was also lengthened. *(83)*

## TURMERIC (Curcuma Longa)

If there's one common kitchen ingredient that you should add to your anti-cancer diet today, its turmeric. This yellow culinary root has been the most clinically tested and written about herb for its anti-inflammatory and anticancer properties. These ground breaking studies found that turmeric might just be one of the most effective common ingredients in the world for keeping you healthy and cancer-free.

For the last 6,000 years traditional Chinese and Ayurvedic medical practitioners prescribed turmeric to alleviate pain, balance digestion, fix liver disorders, purify the blood and clear the skin. Today there is now extensive scientific evidence backing the rationale for its traditional uses including its cancer-fighting properties. Results indicate that the active constituent curcumin, a bright yellow pigment that gives turmeric its yellow colour can inhibit cancer at every stage of its development.

For instance laboratory results have found that curcumin:

- Increases the production and activity of the carcingoen - detoxifying enzyme glutathione - S – transferase.
- Inhibits an enzyme called Cox-2 that promotes inflammation, which as you now know fuels cancer proliferation and spread.
- Inhibits the mTOR pathway, a cell signaling mechanism that plays a critical role in the transformation of healthy cells into cancer cells.
- Inhibits a molecule called NFKB, which is responsible for activating a number of genes that control cancer cells. Even in low concentrations curcumin is a potent inhibitor of NFKB.
- Induces apoptosis, the self-destruct mechanism inherent in normal cells but disabled in cancer cells; causing cancer cells to commit suicide.
- Two other methods by which curcumin can kill cancer cells, is by up-regulating AUTOPHAGY - where cancer cells are cannibalized, and MITOTIC CATASTROPHE - where the cancer cell is destroyed during the process of cell divison.
- Prevents angiogenesis - the growth of new blood vessels that support the growth of tumours
- Increases the antioxidant capacity of the body thereby reducing free radical levels that would otherwise cause cellular damage and could lead to cancer development.

So, as you can see: turmeric/curcumin unlike most anticancer supplements and drugs has been shown to inhibit cancer at every stage i.e. - transformation, initiation, promotion, invasion, angiogenesis and metastasis.[84] Cancers tend to develop over years or even decades, and this Indian spice can halt the process at any of these stages, which is a very remarkable property. Dr. Russell Blaylock, a renowned American Neurosurgeon and author on his musings about turmeric states:

*"There is a multilevel anticancer process that occurs affecting the growth of cancer cells from the use of this Eastern delicacy: Additionally, it strengthens the immune system, lowers blood sugar, and acts as a powerful anti-inflammatory."*

# Studies

Study after study provides strong evidence that the herb turmeric along with its most active constituent curcumin stops many different types of cancer:

- A Chinese study at Zhejian Provincial People's Hospital in 2012 found that curcumin induces cell death in triple-negative breast cancer. This is considered the most aggressive form of breast cancer. *(85)*
- A 2013 study at the University of North Texas Health Science Center found that curcumin suppresses pancreatic cancer tumour growth. *(86)*
- UCLA researchers found in 2011 that curcumin activates cancer-fighting enzymes in patients with head and neck cancers.*(87)*
- A 2006 study published in the journal Neuroscience letters found that curcumin induces cell death in glioblastoma (Brain cancer) cells. *(88)* Curcumin also protects the brain against the harmful side effects of chemotherapy and radiation. This is especially important as chemotherapy is well known to cause significant brain damage (aka, 'chemo-brain') that can lead to poor memory recall and learning difficulties.

## Turmeric (Curcumin) Improves Allopathic Cancer Treatments

Most cancers being treated with chemotherapy drugs will eventually develop "multidrug resistance" in which the cancer cells become immune to the drugs. The cancer cell does this by ejecting the chemotherapy drug from the cell before it can do any harm. Incredibly, curcumin has been shown to reverse this process making previously resistant cancer cells now vulnerable to chemotherapy drugs. In addition, other studies have shown that curcumin not only enhances the effectiveness of radiation treatment against cancer, but also protects surrounding normal tissue within the treatment zone. *(89)*

Some examples of where curcumin has been found to improve the efficiency of allopathic drugs include:

- A German study on colon cancer patients *(90)*
- A leukaemia study found that by combining the anti-leukaemic drug busulfan with curcumin produced synergistic cancer killing that was far greater than the chemotherapy drug alone. *(91)*
- Curcumin was found to improve the efficiency of the drug cisplatin against lung cancer. *(92)*
- Enhancement of allopathic treatments by adding curcumin has also been demonstrated for breast cancer.*(93)*

As researchers keep looking, they continue to find that curcumin can reverse anti-cancer drug resistance in many types of tumours. *(94)*

With all this evidence (and this is by no means a complete list) you may be wondering why curcumin isn't widely prescribed for the prevention and treatment of cancer. The problem is, there is little profit motive. Turmeric and curcumin supplements that come from it are cheap. There's relatively little money to be made but cancer drugs makes pharmaceutical companies and their oncologist salesmen rich beyond their wildest dreams....

## How to take Curcumin

Indians get curcumin by eating turmeric at almost every meal. Most Westerners are not willing to do this. That's why for most of us curcumin supplements are the best option. It's also important that you take the right form. Curcumin by itself is not easily absorbed by the body. Fat increases bioavailability. Fortunately, there are now a number of new formulations designed to be better absorbed.

In addition mixing curcumin powder with extra virgin olive oil or coconut oil and adding a pinch of black pepper can greatly improve absorption. Be careful the mixture can stain everything bright yellow.

Many researchers suggest that we need between 1000 and 4000 mgs of curcumin daily to see any therapeutic effect. Since it would be difficult to consume this level in the spice form, it is advisable to also take curcumin as a supplement.

Doses vary with condition. For cancer prevention, 250mg twice a day should be sufficient. For early cancer 500mg three times a day with meals is sufficient. For metastatic, advanced cancer and very aggressive cancers, the dose can be as high as 2,000mg three times a day. Taking curcumin with food will generally reduce the risk of upset stomach.

*Note:* You should consult your physician before taking high doses of curcumin. It is safe for just about everyone, however, people taking blood thinners such as warfarin or aspirin should exercise some caution. Curcumin is not a blood thinner itself but it can increase the effect of warfarin and other similar drugs.

# ESSIAC TEA

In the 1920s a Canadian nurse named Rene Caisse introduced a herbal tea blended from four different herbs that showed great promise in the treatment of cancer. She named the tea Essiac which is her surname spelt backwards, and used it to successfully treat thousands of patients until her death in 1978 at the age of 90.

Rene first heard about this tea in 1922 while nursing an elderly English woman whose breast was strangely scarred. The woman explained to nurse Caisse that thirty years earlier she was diagnosed with advanced breast cancer and was offered radical mastectomy surgical removal of the breast) as a treatment. Remembering a female friend of hers with similar breast cancer and who went down the mastectomy route but unfortunately didn't survive, the English lady declined this treatment option. Luckily though, she had the good fortune to meet an old Indian medicine man who told her that he could cure her cancer with a "holy tea that would purify her body and place it back in balance with the Great Spirit." (95)

She took up his offer and so, under the medicine man's guidance she drank this pleasant-tasting herbal tea twice daily. He also told her the names of the four herbs used in the tea, and instructed her on its preparation. She was soon healed of her cancer and now thirty years later, at the age of eighty she never had a recurrence. *(96)*

Her story intrigued Rene and so she asked the English lady for the formula. Nurse Caisse in her own words later wrote: "I was much interested and wrote down the names of the herbs she had used. I knew that doctors threw up their hands when cancer was discovered in a patient; it was the same as the death sentence, just about. I decided that if I should ever develop cancer, I would use this herbal tea." *(97)*

About a year after obtaining the herbal recipe, Caisse was visiting a retired doctor who was a friend of hers. As they were walking in his garden, he pointed to a weed and stated: "Nurse Caisse, if people would use this weed there would be very little cancer in the world." *(97)* The weed in question turned out to be sheep sorrel, one of the herbal ingredients in the Indian medicine man's tea.

A few months after that visit, Rene received word that her aunt was diagnosed with stomach cancer and was given only a few months to live. As her condition was terminal the medical profession had nothing it could offer her. So Rene decided to try her herbal tea with her aunts' permission. She set about gathering the herbs and brewed the tea according to the medicine man's instructions. After two months of daily consumption of this brew her aunt was cured. According to Caisse, "My aunt lived for 21 years after being given up on, by the medical profession. There was no recurrence of her cancer." *(97)*

Rene achieved similar success some years later when she administered the Essiac tea to her mum who was diagnosed with terminal inoperable liver cancer and given only days to live. Her mother subsequently recovered and lived without cancer for another 18 years.*(98)*

Over the following years Rene treated thousands of cancer patients using her herbal tea. She recorded many impressive case histories attesting to its efficacy and safety. Although she had clinical x-rays and pathology results proving her remarkable cancer success stories, the Canadian government never officially approved her treatment. Instead, with relentless pressure from the Medical Establishment bearing down on the Ministry of Health, the government of the day threatened to jail her for practicing medicine without a licence. However this created uproar amongst the general public and so a petition with more than 55,000 signatures were collected on her behalf to allow her to continue her work.

For the remainder of her life Rene treated in excess of 40,000 cancer patients, most of them suffering from advanced stages of cancer, having been given up on by the medical profession, as a lost cause.

In that time she refined and perfected the herbal formula in terms of its proportions until she was satisfied she had the optimum medicine to benefit cancer clients. She also worked with many eminent doctors in both Canada and the US, treating their patients. These doctors supervised her work and documented all these cancer patients' results.

Several doctors also visited Nurse Caisse's clinic to ascertain if Essiac really worked. Dr Emma Carson visited her Ottawa clinic in 1937 to review 400 cases of cancer patients who had been treated with Essiac. After reviewing all these cases, Dr Carson declared, "I could scarcely believe my brain and eyes were not deceiving me on some of the most seriously affected cases. The vast majority of Miss Caisse's patients are brought to her for treatment after surgery, radium, x-rays etc had failed to be helpful, and the patients are pronounced incurable. Really, the progress obtainable and the actual results from Essiac treatments and the rapidity of repair were absolutely marvellous and must be seen to convincingly confirm belief."(99)

Among the most compelling anecodotal success stories was the case of Dr. Charles Brusch, one of the most respected physicians in the United States and personal doctor to President John F. Kennedy. In 1984 Dr. Busch was to give Essiac his ultimate vote of confidence after successfully treating his own colorectal cancer solely with Essiac. He signed a notarized statement testifying that he fully endorsed Essiac: *"For I have in fact cured my own cancer, the original site of which was the lower bowel through Essiac alone."*(95)

# THE ESSIAC FORMULA

After more than fifty years of experimentation with various herb combinations and ratios, Rene Caisse settled on her final formula as detailed below that got the best therapeutic results. As she often stated: "If it works, don't change it." The herbs that are used to make the authentic Essiac tea are:

- Burdock root (chopped into small pea-sized pieces)
- Powered sheep sorrel (whole plant ie. roots and leaves)
- Powered slippery elm inner bark
- Powered turkey rhubarb root

In the correct combination, these herbs strengthen the immune system; reduce the toxic side-effects of pharmaceutical drugs; reduce inflammation; increase energy levels and have anti-cancer properties.(95) "Essiac is by its very nature non-toxic" wrote Thomas. "And therein lays its real power. Essiac is the ultimate body purifier. Thus, the body once it is cleansed of toxic disease producing impurities has the power to heal itself." (95) In his books, 'Cancer therapy', and 'Herbs against cancer', Dr Ralph Moss cites studies where each of the herbs in Essiac have been shown to demonstrate a significant amount of anticancer activity (100, 101) A good source of information on Essiac is: 'The alternative Cancer Care' website (102) which has many research studies about the healing power of Essiac tea. And to get the full story about its history check out the Health Freedom Network website.(103)

These four herbs are thoroughly mixed together in corresponding ratios of 24:16:4:1

For example:

Burdock - 24 grams

Sheep Sorrel - 16 grams

Slippery elm - 4 grams

Thurkey rhubarb - 1 gram

Total weight 45 grams

- To make the tea, put the herb mixture in a large stainless steel pot and add in purified water (ratio of herb mix to water is 1:32 ie. 45 grams: (45 x 32 ml) = 1.44 litres of water
- Cover the pot with its lid, bring to boil and continue boiling hard for ten minutes. Turn off the heat and leave the pot sitting on the warm plate for approximately twelve hours with its lid on.
- After twelve hours reheat the brew until steaming hot, but not boiling and allow it to settle for a few minutes.
- Then strain the hot liquid through a fine strainer into waiting hot sterilized bottles and immediately seal the bottles. When the bottles cool they can be stored in the fridge if you have space for them, or they can be stored in a cool dark cupboard. Once opened Essiac tea must then be stored in the fridge since there are no preservatives in the recipe.

## How to take Essiac tea

Pour 30 ml of Essiac tea into 60 ml of hot water and sip it once daily. The best time to drink Essiac is before bedtime on an empty stomach (ie. at least 2 hours after eating). This tea can be consumed long-term however it is recommended to take it for three weeks in a row then abstain for the fourth week in order to stimulate maximum efficacy of the tea.

Rene Caisse considered it important not to increase the 30ml dosage as it provided no additional benefit but could risk the possibility of stimulating over detoxification, in other words, the patient could experience a classic 'Herxheimer Reaction'.

## THE BOTTOM LINE

I imagine the million dollar question on everyone's mind is if Essiac tea is the closest thing to the proverbial magic bullet for curing cancer! There is no doubt that thousands of people have claimed to have been brought back from the brink of death by Rene Caisse's tea. Caisse herself stated that Essiac caused regression in tumours, prolonged life, relieved pain, and in the right circumstances with patients whose organs weren't already destroyed, could cure cancer. *(104)*

It is well known that this tea has remarkable detoxifying properties and it gives a great boost to the immune system, two characteristics that can help the cancer sufferer on the road to recovery.

Dr. Keith Block, a well regarded oncologist who uses natural remedies in his medical practice regards Essiac as a *"weak combination of anticancer herbs"*.*(105)* John Boik, a cancer researcher, who identified a number of natural compounds, with anticancer activity agrees that Essiac does indeed contain certain compounds with anti-tumour properties, however, he believes such compounds need to be taken in far greater amounts than what the Essiac tea affords. *(106)*

So, is it possible that Essiac is less effective for today's cancer patients, than it was in Caisse's heyday? In those times, their diet and environment were less polluted than those of today's cancer patients. In addition, today's patients have probably received high dose chemotherapy and radiation treatments. All of this places an even greater burden on the cancer patients immune and detoxification systems, making the regression of cancer a more difficult task.

So in light of this, it is my recommendation that Essiac tea should be used in conjunction with all the other therapies described in this book to effect a favourable outcome in the battle against cancer.


## THE HOXSEY HERBAL TONIC

For nearly 40 years Harry Hoxsey (1901-1974) a self-taught healer with no medical training, treated and reputedly cured many cancer patients including the terminally ill using an herbal tonic and/or salve, which he claimed had been handed down by his great-grandfather. *(107)*

The story goes that Hoxsey's great grandfather had a horse that was cured of a leg tumour after grazing on some wild flowers and herbs. His great-grandfather then formulated these botanicals into an herbal tonic and salve and used them to treat other horses.

Harry's father who was a veterinarian, also used the ointment and tonic to treat cancerous growths on animals (and sometimes humans too). He passed the formula to his son Harry while lying on his deathbed with the proviso that the formula was not to be used primarily for monetary gain, but to allow its use for as many cancer victims as possible.

Word soon spread about Harry's miracle cancer cure, and he became locally known as 'The Cancer Doctor'. In 1924 Harry went to Chicago to demonstrate his treatment on a terminally ill policeman, Sgt. Thomas Manix, using both the ointment and tonic, Sgt Manix was completely cured. The doctors were so impressed that they offered to buy the formula from Hoxsey. Hoxsey didn't like their terms and so refused to hand over the formula. This enraged the doctors who were closely affilated with the American Medical Association (AMA) and so began a 40 year battle with the medical establishment to denounce him as a fraud. *(108)*

Despite constant harassment from the medical establishment and law enforcement agencies, Hoxsey managed to operate a chain of cancer clinics throughout 17 states in the USA. He had the largest chain of privately owned cancer treatment centres at the time. But in the 1950's all of Hoxsey's clinics were shut down, even though a 1953 Federal Report to the Senate found that the American Medical Association (AMA), the Food and Drug Administration (FDA) and the National Cancer Institute (NCI) had organised a "conspiracy to suppress a fair, unbiased assessment of Hoxsey's methods" (The Fitzgerald Report) *(109)*

Despite the ongoing harassment Harry's cancer treatment received the endorsement of many prominent doctors, senators and even two federal judges upheld the "therapeutic value" of Hoxsey's tonic. Even his arch-enemies the AMA and the FDA were forced to admit that his treatment could cure some forms of cancer. The Assistant District Attorney of Dallas, Al Templeton arrested Harry almost 100 times until his brother Mike Templeton developed cancer that was considered incurable by conventional medicine, but when he received treatment at Hoxsey's clinic he made a full recovery. The assistant DA credited his brother's cure to Hoxsey's treatment and for a time he also became

Hoxsey's lawyer.

Esquire magazine sent journalist James Burke to Hoxsey's Dallas cancer clinic in 1939 to expose the presumed quack. Burke spent six weeks there, talking to patients and investigating the whole set up. During that time he became convinced the Hoxsey's clinic was actually curing cancer. Burke wrote an article entitled "The Quack who Cures Cancer." *(110)* However Esquire wouldn't publish it because it didn't suit their agenda! Burke subsequently worked for Hoxsey as a press agent.

In 1954 an independent team of 10 US doctors spent two days examining patient records in Hoxsey's Dallas clinic, and concluded that he was successfully treating pathologically proven cases of cancer, both internal and external without the use of conventional means.

For thirty years he kept his cancer formula a closely guarded secret until the FDA used the courts to demand ingredient labeling. Hoxsey finally agreed to the courts demand that he make public his formula. He listed a core set of his ingredients as a base with various other herbs added, depending upon the individual cancer cases being treated. In his 1956 autobiographical book, "You Don't Have To Die", *(107)* Hoxsey lists the ingredients in his herbal tonic, given in "all cases of cancer, both internal and external", as potassium iodide combined with some or all of the following herbs on a case-by-case basis:

- Liquorice (Glycyrrhiza glabra)
- Red clover (Trifolouim protense)
- Burdock root (Arctium lappa)
- Stillingia root (Stillingia sylvatica)
- Barberry bark (Berberis vulgaris)
- Poke root (Phytolacca americana)
- Cascara (Rhamnus purshiana)
- Prickly Ash bark (Zanithoxylum americanum)
- Buck thorn bark (Rhamnus catharticus)

The external treatment is a paste, which is applied to skin cancers. It's a mixture of bloodroot, zinc oxide and antimony sulfide.

Hoxsey considered cancer to be a systemic disease however

localised its manifestation might appear to be. He believed his herbal concoction detoxified the body, balanced body chemistry and allowed the body to digest and excrete tumours.

A lady by the name of Mildred Nelson who was Hoxsey's long term assistant was first introduced to the Hoxsey method when her mother sought him out for treatment for her cancer. Mildred a conventionally trained nurse believed Hoxsey to be a charlaton and she tried to talk her mother out of such quackery. Instead she ended up taking a job at Hoxsey's clinic as a nurse when her mother recovered fully from the cancer. In a 1984 interview Nelson gave her views on the efficacy of the Hoxsey tonic. She believes it "normalizes and balances the chemistry within the body. When you get everything normalized, the abnormal cells (ie. tumour cells) cease to grow. And very slowly the tumour is absorbed and excreted and it's gone." *(111)*

Although both the AMA and FDA dismissed the Hoxsey potion as "worthless, without any therapeutic merit in the treatment of cancer," in the years since then medical literature has discovered anti-cancer substances in virtually all "Hoxsey's herbs."

According to botanist James A Duke of the United States Dept. of Agriculture, eight of the nine Hoxsey-tonic herbs have some anti-tumour activity in animal models, five have antioxidant effects and all nine have antimicrobial activity that may be linked to cancer-fighting effects. Duke's assessment was that the Hoxsey tonic ingredients showed very significant anti-cancer activity. *(112)*

Medical historian Patricia Spain Ward PhD reported "provocative findings of anti-tumour properties" in many of the individual Hoxsey herbs when she was commissioned to investigate the Hoxsey regimen in 1988 for the United States Congress. *(113)*

Today, the Hoxsey therapy is still practiced at the Bio-Medical Centre in Tijuana, Mexico, combined with nutritional supplements and specific dietary restrictions. *(114)* Patients are expected to exclude certain foods from their diet that nullify the tonic, such as pork, processed flour, tomatoes, alcohol, carbonated drinks and vinegar.

---
**CHAPTER 8**
---

# TREATING CANCER WITH ESSENTIAL OILS

*"And the leaves of the tree are for the healing of the nations."* (Revelation 22:2)

**E**ssential oils (EO's) are volatile organic compounds extracted from medicinal plants that carry the essence of the plant in such a potent form that a single drop can equal multiple teaspoons of the plant in its dried form. For instance, one drop of peppermint oil is equivalent to 25 cups of peppermint tea.

EO's can be extracted from plant leaves, flower stems, roots or bark. EO's are collected when the plant matter is hydro-distilled, in other words, hot steam is sent through the plant, separating the volatile oil compounds from the plant material. The chemical composition for an individual EO varies based on growing conditions of the plant and from which part of the plant it was derived.

EO's have been used for thousands of years in Eastern medicine, Ayurvedic medicine and Chinese medicine. They have been referenced more than 300 times in the bible. People have derived numerous benefits from these oil extracts for centuries due to their antibacterial, antimicrobial, antiviral, antiseptic, antibiotic and anti-inflammatory properties. Now researchers are discovering that many EO's possess anticancer properties, and that these oils can help not only prevent, but treat cancer and its debilitating side-effects. Most research to this point has been conducted in the laboratory (i.e., in vitro) and results suggest that many different chemical constituents of EO's have anticancer properties. *(1)* And although we do not have any major human studies with hundreds or thousands of participants to verify these discoveries; a quick check on the internet will bring up thousands upon thousands of testimonials of people claiming that EO's helped cure them of cancer. These stories are not to be scoffed at, especially when you consider the vast majority of these individuals share their story with no ulterior motive such as monetary gain.

## ESSENTIAL OIL CHARACTERISTICS

Over 300 different compounds have been identified in EO's, which have been classified into three main groups:

- Terpenes and terpenoids
- Phenolic compounds
- Alkane and Alkene compounds

Both the terpene group and the phenolic group of compounds are found in abundance in EO's and in a lower extent the alkane and alkene compounds in trace amounts. *(1)* All of these compounds are characterised by a low molecular weight; meaning they can be as much as a thousand times smaller than say, an olive oil or a coconut oil compound. That means that the great thing about EO's is that they are transdermal, meaning they can pass easily through the skin. They can also quickly enter your body through inhalation. Another incredible thing is that many EO compounds can pass through the blood-brain barrier due to their tiny molecular weight.

You can also ingest EO's where they quickly enter the blood stream to be distributed around the body. A word of caution though – not all EO's can by used internally and not everyone is able to use them this way. Oils high in phenols, such as oregano, thyme and cinnamon are generally more likely to accumulate in the liver if it is anyway compromised. Use such oils with care. As a general guideline, the hotter the oil, the more precaution is necessary.

# BEST ESSENTIAL OILS FOR CANCER PATIENTS

There are many ways that EO's can help in cancer healing including emotional healing, stress relief and detoxification. However, some well researched EO's are shown to act directly and indirectly on cancer cells, preventing their growth by stopping angiogenesis or even promoting apoptosis (cancer cell death). It is believed that virtually all EO's possess anticancer properties, but the following is a list of some of the most important EO's that show the most promise in the prevention and treatment of cancer.

# FRANKINCENSE

There are those who contend that Frankincense is the king of the EO's when it comes to healing properties. Frankincense essential oil is obtained by hydro distillation of the Boswellia species gum resins derived from the bark of the Boswellia tree. It has a long history in myth and folk medicine. It is mentioned in the Bible where it is one of the three gifts offered to the baby Jesus by the wise men (possibly because of its healing powers). In the Middle East, where it originates, frankincense has been used for religious purposes for centuries and is a part component of their holy anointing oil, which also contains myrrh essential oil; the second gift offered to Jesus by the wise men.

Frankincense essential oil contains boswellic acid, which has strong anti-inflammatory activity. This has important implications in the fight against cancer as numerous studies have linked inflammation to cancer. By disrupting inflammatory processes, frankincense could stop cancer before it starts!

A 2006 study published in Planta Medica uncovered a number of ways the boswellic acid in frankincense might fight inflammatory diseases and cancer. The study showed that boswellic acid inhibited 5-lipoxygenase, an enzyme involved in inflammatory processes. (2) The researchers also found that boswellic acid might target free radicals and cytokines. Both of these play a role in inflammation.

Some evidence also suggests that frankincense might target cancer cells without harming healthy cells. A 2009 study of bladder cancer, studied how frankincense affected cultures of normal and cancerous bladder cells. The oil attacked cancerous cells vigorously via multiple pathways, but it did not harm healthy cells. (3)

A 2015 study found similar effects in breast cancer. The researchers found that frankincense could kill breast cancer cells and disrupt the growth of future cancer cells. (4)

When frankincense was tested against human pancreatic cancer cells, it was able to cause substantial levels of cancer cell death by inhibiting signalling molecules and cell cycle regulators. The constituent in frankincense oil responsible for this destructive power is "beta-elemene". (5)

Not only has frankincense oil been seen to have cytotoxic (cancer killing) activity, it was recently demonstrated to be, "As effective as the common cancer treatment drugs doxorubicin and 5-flourouracil in treating cancer. (6)

Just to show how powerful frankincense EO can be, researchers at the University of Oklahoma Health Science Centre confirmed that one man used it to cure basal cell carcinoma on his arm. Just by applying frankincense oil to the cancer every day for twenty weeks, and he didn't experience any side effects. (7)

One of the most amazing things about frankincense is that its essential oils are very, very small molecular compounds. These compounds are so small, they can actually pass through the blood-brain barrier and start to reduce inflammation in the brain as well as attack and kill brain tumours. For example, many brain cancer patients experience cerebral oedema (swelling in the head) after their tumours have been surgically removed, or after radiation therapy. This is usually treated with steroids, which can cause more side effects. A 2011 study found that frankincense EO can offer a much safer alternative to this medication. *(8)* In the study 60% of patients had their swelling reduced by 75% or more.

Other health benefits of frankincense EO include:

- Boosting of immunity
- Destruction of toxins and candida overgrowth
- Relief of arthritic pain
- Aid to digestion
- Balance of hormones
- Improvement of skin health
- Provision of neurological support*(9)*

Since frankincense oil is so good at calming and de-stressing the mind, this in itself will do immense good as a soothing agent for all cancer cases. Because frankincense has so many health-promoting properties, is it no wonder that it is often referred to as the "Oil of Kings" and "Liquid Gold".

## Directions for using Frankincense EO

The benefits of frankincense EO can be acquired by inhaling it, applying it topically on the skin, or ingesting it in very small amounts (1-2 drops). For example, you can rub a few drops of this EO on your neck area, especially at the sides where the lymphatic nodes are located, and do this three times daily.

Frankincense EO can also be blended with other carrier oil such as coconut, jojoba or sweet almond oil and the mixture rubbed all over the body.

You can also take one to two drops internally either diluted in 100ml of water or a liquid such as coconut or almond milk or you can put a drop or two under your tongue or apply it to the roof of your mouth (especially good for those who have brain cancer).

Frankincense oil can also be used in diffusers (preferably cold mist diffusers) or directly inhaled from the bottle for a few deep breaths.

# MYRRH

Native to regions in Africa and the Middle East, the species commiphora myrrha, is a small tree that produces a sap that hardens into a resin known as myrrh. Through a process using steam distillation myrrh resin is converted into an essential oil with a dry, woody aroma.

Myrrh is mentioned in the Bible over 160 times as it is one of the precious gifts (together with gold and frankincense) offered by the three wise men to the new-born baby Jesus. Like frankincense, myrrh is also listed as an ingredient in the holy anointing oil used to anoint the tabernacle high priests and kings.

Myrrh has been used throughout history as a perfume, incense, and health aid. It has powerful cleansing properties, and both the resin and essential oil are valued for their wound-healing properties. Maintaining healthy skin is one of myrrh oil's renowned uses as it helps restore the health of skin cells thereby reducing the appearance of wrinkles.

Myrrh has antibacterial properties and it is a specific and highly effective antiseptic astringent for inflammation and infections of the mouth, throat and gums. It is a common ingredient in herbal tooth paste and mouthwashes.

Other benefits of myrrh, includes improved digestion. Its antibacterial and antifungal properties help kill off candida overgrowth and other pathogenic factors in the gut. The scientific studies that have been carried out on myrrh have proven that its health benefits can be attributed to its powerful antioxidant, antifungal, antiviral, anti-inflammatory, anti parasitic, expectorant, antispasmodic and yes anti-cancer properties.*(10)*

There are many health enhancing compounds in myrrh EO, two of the most active being terpenoids and sesquiterpenes. Terpenoids have powerful antioxidant properties that help reduce inflammation in the body, (a major promoter of cancer growth) while sesquiterpenes, because of their small molecular size, have the ability to cross the blood-brain barrier where they can affect certain parts of your brain, particularly your hypothalamus, pituitary and the limbic system (your emotional centre) which brings about a calming and balancing effect on your emotions and nervous system.

The role that myrrh EO plays in cancer therapies is becoming a hot topic among cancer researchers in recent times. Among its medicinal uses just outlined, myrrh EO has demonstrated notable cancer killing abilities. A good example is in a study published in Phytotherapy Research in March 2016 where Welsh researchers found that a phytochemical from myrrh EO known as beta-bisabolene showed cancer-killing activity against four lines of human breast cancer cells.*(11)* Amongst these are triple negative and HER2 positive breast cancers, both of which tend to be more aggressive forms of breast cancer.

Another study conducted by Chinese researchers, published in April 2011 issue of the Journal of Medicinal Plants Research, also found that extracts made from myrrh resin were able to reduce the proliferation or replication of human cancer cells. They found that myrrh inhibited growth in eight different types of cancer cells, specifically gynaecological cancers. *(12)*

Another very interesting study came out of China in 2013 where myrrh and frankincense were both studied in combination to assess their cancer fighting abilities. They studied the effects of the two EO's independently and as a mixture, on five different tumour cell lines. The results indicated that two cell lines showed increased sensitivity to the myrrh and frankincense EO's compared with the remaining cell lines. In addition, the anticancer effects of myrrh were markedly increased compared with those of frankincense. *(13)*

My recommendation is for you to use both frankincense and myrrh

EO's together for their synergistic blend of anti-inflammatory, antimicrobial and anticancer benefits. Notably, these two EO's are generally prescribed together in traditional Chinese medicine.

## Directions for using Myrrh EO's

- Diffuse or inhale it.

  You can diffuse several drops of myrrh into the room you are sitting in by using a cool mist diffuser. It is better not to heat EO's as this may damage their therapeutic effects. You can also directly inhale the aromas directly from the bottle, or just place a couple of drops of oil into your hands and place them over your nose and mouth and breathe in deeply for a minute or two.

- Apply it directly to the skin.

  It is best to dilute myrrh EO with a carrier oil such as coconut, jojoba or almond oil before applying it to the skin. You can also add a few drops to your shampoo and cosmetic products, or enjoy a healing bath by placing a few drops along with a cup of Epsom salts in your bath.

- Taking it internally

  Dilute one drop in 100ml of liquid such as coconut or rice milk.

# LAVENDER

Lavender essential oil comes for lavender angustifolia, an easy-to-grow evergreen shrub that produces clumps of beautiful purple scented flowers. High quality lavender oil has a sweet, floral and slightly woody scent. Its colour can range from pale yellow to yellow-green and it can also be colourless. Both lavender and its essential oil are valued for their fragrance and medicinal qualities. The flowers are used for potpourris, while the essential oil is added to bath and body-care products such as shampoos, soaps, perfumes and household cleaning products. It is one of the most used and well known oils in aromatherapy, especially for its calming and relaxing properties which can aid in distress, anxiety, insomnia, depression and pain relief. *(14)* Its effectiveness is believed to be due to the physiological effects of its volatile oils on the limbic (emotional) system within the brain.

Lavender essential oil is also known for its anti-inflammatory, antiseptic, antibacterial, antiviral, antifungal and antimicrobial properties.

## Biochemistry of Lavender EO's

Lavender EO has a chemically complex structure with over 150 active constituents. This oil is rich in esters which are aromatic molecules with antispasmodic (stopping spasms and pain) calming and relaxing properties. *(15)* The chief botanical constituents of lavender EO are linalylacetate, linalool, terpinen-4-ol and camphor. Other constituents in lavender oil that are responsible for its antimicrobial and anti-inflammatory properties include cis-ocimene, lavandulylacetate, 1,8-cineole, limonene and geraniol.

## Lavender's Benefits for Cancer Patients

There has been significant research on lavender's influence on cancer, with studies demonstrating its anti-tumoural properties. It has been shown to reduce the size of tumours, inhibit cell growth and reset programmed cell death (apoptosis) in cancer cells. *(16)* One of the active phytochemicals within lavender is linalool. Research in 2016 indicated it had significant cytotoxic (cancer cell killing) and apoptotic (programmed cell death) activity against epithelial ovarian cancer cells. In addition, researchers found that combining linalool with the chemotherapy agent paclitaxel significantly decreased tumour weight, compared with the use of paclitaxel alone. *(17)*

2015 research on linalool against human melanoma cells revealed that linalool had an inhibitory effect on the growth of these cells. *(18)*

A 2014 study demonstrated that lavender essential oil exhibited strong cytotoxic effects against malignant cervical cancer cells. *(19)* It also had the same effect on both oestrogen and progesterone-receptor positive breast cancer cells.

In another study from 2013, researchers found that lavender decreased the viability of Hodgkin's lymphoma cells. *(20)* It did this by inhibiting cell proliferation (rapid growth) and by inducing apoptosis in the cancer cells.

Research in 2015 found that perillylalcohol, a constituent of lavender, when administered via nasal inhalation, was an effective treatment for glioblastoma (a type of brain cancer) patients. *(21)* These patients had become unresponsive to chemo and radiation, but lived several years longer while inhaling the perillylalcohol with no adverse side effects.

In other research, Chinese scientists observed that lavender essential oil can upregulate levels of the body's antioxidant enzymes; catalase, glutathione peroxidise and superoxide dismutase. *(22)* Romanian researchers noted similar activity by simply inhaling lavender for an hour each day. *(23)* Considering that these enzymes are responsible for quenching free radicals thereby reducing inflammation within the body, any means of upregulating their activity is highly welcomed in the treatment of cancer or any chronic illness.

## How to use Lavender EO

- Put a few drops of lavender EO into your hands, rub hands together and deeply inhale the scent for a minute or two to enjoy its calming effects.
- Lavender EO can also be diffused into the room using a cool mist diffuser. As with all essential oils never heat them as it ruins their therapeutic properties.
- It can be applied directly to the skin where it's absorbed into the bloodstream within 20 minutes. To heal cuts, burns or abrasions it's recommended to dilute it in a carrier oil.

On a last note: make sure lavender essential oil is derived from true lavender, "Lavandula angustifolia" and not lavandin. Lavandin is often substituted by makers of cheaper essential oils because it yields more oil than true lavender. Lavandin is not a legitimate substitute for lavandula angustifolia as it does not possess the same healing properties and should never be used on burns.

# LEMONGRASS

Lemongrass essential oil is extracted from the leaves of the Cymbopogon species of plants. This plant grows in dense clumps and has bright green sharp-edged leaves similar to grass. *(24)* Lemongrass EO has a thin consistency and a pale or bright yellow colour. It has a strong, fresh, lemony and earthy scent.

Lemongrass is a popular flavouring in Asian cooking, added to curries and soups. It is also suitable for poultry, beef and fish. Fresh lemongrass is also used to make a refreshing lemony flavoured herbal tea.

## Health Properties

Lemongrass is loaded with a wide variety of medicinal compounds that exhibit properties such as;

- Anti-bacterial
- Anti-fungal
- Anti-parasitic
- Antioxidant
- Anti-inflammatory
- Detoxifying *(25)*

These compounds include a diverse array of terpenes, ketones, esters, flavonoids and phenols. Citral, a chemical compound present in lemongrass that gives it a lemony aroma and taste, exhibits anticancer activity. *(26)* A drink with as little as one gram of lemongrass contains enough citral to prompt cancer cells to commit suicide by causing apoptosis (self-destruction) says a 2005 study reported in Planta Med. *(27)*

Researchers in India conducted a study to find out how lemongrass extract interacted with two different cancer cell lines commonly used in cancer research, which were both cervical cancer cell strains. The tests involved using lemongrass oil and citral emulsion, the same compound found in lemongrass. In the study lemongrass oil and citral emulsion both had significant effects, such as preventing the proliferation or spread of the cancer cells while also inducing apoptosis. The study's abstract ends with the authors conclusion that; "All the results suggest lemongrass oil and citral emulsion could be considered as potent candidates for anticancer agents." *(28)*

A 2009 study was published that evaluated the essential oil from a lemongrass variety of Cymbopogon flexuous for its in vitro (using Petridish specimens) cytotoxicity against 12 different human cancer cell lines; as well as in vivo (using a live animal) anticancer effects on mice. The results were quite remarkable. The animal trials showed that direct injection of lemongrass EO inhibited cancer tumours in a dose-dependent way, meaning the higher the dose, the better the results. *(29)*

During their research, they discovered that the EO triggers a variety of mechanisms that kill cancer cells. They conclude by stating; "Our results indicate that the oil has a promising anticancer activity and causes loss in tumour cell viability by activating the apoptotic process as identified by electron microscopy."

A more recent in vitro study published in the journal Pharmacognosy Communications in 2013 reveals that lemongrass was also effective against cervical cancer. Researchers found that lemongrass not only stopped cervical cancer cells (as well as several other types of cancer cells) from spreading, but it also initiated cancer cell apoptosis, also known as programmed cell death. *(30)*

Several more recent in vitro studies on different extracts of lemongrass have all demonstrated varying degrees of cytotoxicity towards cancer cells. *(31)* What's even more exciting is that some of the latest in vitro and in vivo animal studies suggest that it could be at least as effective as chemotherapy in targeting cancer cells, without the harmful toxic effects of chemotherapy.

Now, while these results are exciting and hopeful, it's important to understand that these studies have been completed using either cells in a lab or animal models. No human subjects or cancer patients have undergone trials to see if this effect translates to the human body. But like I keep saying throughout this book, it would be beyond lunacy to just rely on one or two agents to combat this multi-faceted disease we call cancer.

## How to use Lemongrass

There are two main ways to get the benefits of lemongrass in your daily life:

- Lemongrass essential oil
- Lemongrass tea

Lemongrass tea tastes of lemon, but sweeter and less strong, making for a delicious herbal tea. Many people drink this tea for healthy digestion and to support their body's disease-fighting defences. To make lemongrass tea, take two to three stalks of lemongrass and cut off the tough upper stem to find the tender inner flesh. Chop into one-inch pieces. Pour a cup of boiling water over them and steep for 15 minutes. Strain and drink twice daily to reduce your risk of cancer.

Lemongrass essential oil can be used as a fresh citrus seasoning in cooking. You may choose to incorporate it in your curry dishes, in soups or seafood dishes.

To diffuse lemongrass essential oil, put 4-5 drops in a cool mist diffuser to breathe in the aromatic power of this healing oil.

You can also dilute a few drops of lemongrass EO in a carrier oil to use topically.

# OREGANO

Oregano is a common culinary herb native to the Mediterranean region and is part of the mint family. This fragrant herb is commonly used to flavour pasta and meat dishes and can be used in many different recipes.

Oregano essential oil is derived from its shoots, leaves and flowers through steam distillation. It has a number of powerful chemicals, which gives it a strong flavour and also impressive medicinal abilities. This EO is a powerful antimicrobial that can help fight off infection. It also has potent antibacterial, antiviral and antifungal properties. [32] I highly recommend you adding this oil to your arsenal of natural healing tools.

## Cancer-fighting Properties

A few studies have indicated that carvacrol, the most abundant compound in oregano EO inhibits cancer cell growth and causes cell death in lung [33] liver [34] breast [35] colon [36] prostate and skin cancer cell lines. [37]

Another phytochemical in oregano EO, carnosol, has also been evaluated for anticancer properties in prostate, breast, skin, leukaemia and colon cancer with promising results. [36]

In another more recent study researchers have shown that oregano EO kills 99% of human breast cancer cells in vitro at remarkably low concentrations. In fact, they found that oregano was the most powerful of four essential oils (sage, ginseng, stevia) at killing all six different cancer cell lines tested, including cervical, breast, leukaemia, lung and colon cancer. [38]

How? It was discovered that oregano EO almost completely depletes cancer cells of their glutathione - an antioxidant they need to survive. Without glutathione, cancer cells are highly vulnerable to oxidative stress (free radical damage) and quickly die.

## How to use Oregano Oil

Oregano EO can be applied to the skin or taken by mouth, depending on the condition being treated. However, the oil must always be diluted. Here is a guide for how to use it;

- On the skin: For skin conditions or infections, dilute with olive or coconut oil at a concentration of one teaspoon (5ml) of the carrier oil per drop of oregano oil, then apply to the affected area.
- Under the tongue: Dilute with a carrier oil at a ratio of one drop of oregano oil to one drop of the carrier oil. Place 1-3 drops of this dilution under the tongue, hold it there for a few minutes, then flush with water.
- Swallowed: if you're taking oregano oil orally, you can put a few drops of it into a cup of vegetable milk and gargle and then swallow.

# ROSEMARY

Rosemary is a small evergreen plant that belongs to the mint family. Looking similar to lavender, rosemary has leaves like flat pine needles touched with silver. Its leaves are commonly used fresh or dried to flavour culinary dishes. Rosemary essential oil has a clear, refreshing herbal smell, is colourless and has a watery viscosity. It contains some very potent chemical constituents, which are steam distilled from the leaves and flowering tops of the plant.

## Therapeutic qualities of Rosemary EO

According to Modern Essentials, a guide to the therapeutic uses of essential oils, high-quality rosemary oil has analgesic, antibacterial, anticancer, anti-catarrhal, antifungal, anti-infection, anti-inflammatory, antioxidant and expectorant properties. *(39)*

Most of rosemary's beneficial health effects have been attributed to the high antioxidant activity of its main chemical constituents, including carnosol, carnosic acid, limonene, ursolic acid, rosmarinic acid and caffeic acid. *(40)* These potent antioxidants helps protect against oxidative stress and free radicals, which damage cell membranes, tamper with DNA, causing the death of healthy cells and the development of cancerous conditions.

In addition to being a rich antioxidant, rosemary is also known for its anticancer and anti-inflammatory properties. One of rosemary's main active constituents is carnosol. According to an article published in the journal "Cancer Letters" in 2011, "Carnosol has been evaluated for anticancer property in prostate, breast, skin, leukaemia and colon caner with promising results." *(41)*

In addition, carnosol appears to have "a selective toxicity towards cancer cells versus non-tumourigenic cells (ie, healthy cells) and is well tolerated when administered to animals.

Another article published in the journal "Nutrients" in 2016 notes that rosemary extract has demonstrated anticancer properties in the laboratory (in vitro) for the following cancers: colon, liver, lung, breast, prostate, ovarian, cervical, bladder and pancreatic cancers. *(42)*

So, the evidence is there for all to see; with dozens of research studies providing the cancer-killing properties of rosemary essential oil, I strongly encourage you to include this oil in your natural health armoury in the battle against cancer.

## How to use:

To use rosemary essential oil, it can be diffused, inhaled and applied transdermally. Before using it topically, it is recommended you dilute it in a carrier oil, as there is a risk of contact sensitivity. Do a skin patch text first.

You can also use fresh rosemary-infused oil on your salads as a delicious dressing.

# THYME

Thyme is a member of the mint family and has a sweet, earthy flavour that lends itself well to cooking. The EO is derived from steam distillation of fresh thyme flowers and leaves.

Many of thyme's beneficial properties come from its essential oils, which include potent compounds like thymol, camphene, linalool and carvacrol. Thymol which makes up from 20% to more than 50% of thyme EO is known as a biocide, which means it can destroy harmful microorganisms and give thyme oil strong antimicrobial properties. Other volatile compounds of thyme oil, such as camphene and alpha-pinene, are able to strengthen the immune system with their antibacterial and antifungal properties. (43)

This makes them effective both inside and outside the body, protecting the mucous membranes, gut and respiratory system from potential infections. The compound linalool has strong antioxidant properties that help to reduce free radical damage, an initiator of carcinogenesis.

## Anti-Carcinogenic activity of Thyme

The journal Molecules published (2010) a study done in Switzerland that evaluated a number of essential oils against various human cancer cell lines. Included was thyme EO and it stood out as having the strongest cytotoxic effect (i.e., cancer killing) toward all three types of cancer cell lines tested, which were breast, lung, and prostate cancer cells. (44) This is likely due to the active compound thymol, which has been shown to activate a number of cancer-killing mechanisms.

Also, another (2012) study carried out by researchers at Celal Bayar University in Turkey and published in the journal 'Nutrition and Cancer' sought to investigate the effects wild thyme might have on breast cancer cells. The researchers in this study confirmed that wild thyme induced cell death in the breast cancer cells. They noted that in as little as 72 hours of in vitro (i.e., petri dish) breast cancer treatment, thyme essential oil was able to kill 98% of the cancer breast cells with a concentration of only 0.05%. (45)

As one of the primary herbs to facilitate oestrogen binding, thyme EO can also help balance and regulate hormones. *(46)* For women who have breast or ovarian cancers, thyme EO can also act as nature's "Kinder, gentler" forms of Tamoxifen by preventing the more dangerous forms of oestrogen and xynoestrogen compounds from binding to cancer cell receptors, which would otherwise promote cancer growth in those organs. (Taxmoxifen is an oestrogen binder that can be of value in short-term use to slow down breast cancer, but in long-term use, elevates the risk of heart attacks, liver damage and endometrial cancer).

In other studies, the active compound thymol, found in thyme oil, is effective at killing and suppressing stomach cancer cells. *(47)* Thyme EO has been shown to inhibit proliferation of DLD-1 colorectal cancer cells through its powerful antioxidant effect. *(48)*

## Taking Thyme Essential Oil

- As a condiment, put 1-2 drops in meat and fish dishes to add a fresh herbal flavour.

- Dilute 1-2 drops in a carrier oil such as coconut, jojoba or sweet almond oil and apply to the desired area on the skin.

- Dilute 1-2 drops in 100 ml of liquid (i.e., almond, coconut milk, etc.) and drink.

## SOME FINAL THOUGHTS ON ESSENTIAL OILS

Despite their incredible diversity, essential oils seem to have one thing in common; virtually all of them possess anti-cancer properties to one degree or another. Common characteristics shared by most EO's include having antioxidant, antiseptic, antimicrobial and anti-inflammatory properties, which benefit cancer patients greatly.

Another way to appreciate and understand the potency of essential oils is to look into their frequency. You may be surprised to learn that everything in the universe vibrates at a frequency whether it's living creatures, plants or objects. This frequency can be measured in Megahertz (MHZ) and the frequency is defined as "a measureable rate of electrical flow that is constant between any two points."

Essential oils possess some of the highest frequencies that can be found in nature and as such they are able to create an environment that is hostile to disease-causing bacteria, viruses, fungi and more. Their high frequency property makes them an excellent therapeutic tool for fighting many diseases including cancer.

In his book, *"The Body Electric"* Robert O. Becker M.D., finds that people who have their body frequencies in the range of 62 - 78 MHz experience good health. Disease has a frequency that begins at 58 MHz. If certain frequencies are fed into the human body, they may be able to prevent the development of disease while other frequencies can possibly destroy the disease completely. Generally speaking, substances of higher frequency will get rid of diseases of lower frequency. Given that cancer has a frequency of 42 MHz, it is possible that the high frequency of essential oils can halt or prevent this disease. Some example of therapeutic grade essential oil frequencies are as follows:

- Frankincense – 147 MHz

- Lavender – 118MHz

- Myrrh – 105 MHz

When purchasing essential oils I would caution that quality is key. Many essential oils are synthetically produced and diluted with alcohol and other additives. To be effective, only 100% pure therapeutic grade quality essential oils must be used, otherwise you will not obtain the health benefits.

Because essential oils are highly concentrated; it normally takes a few hundred kilos and sometimes a few tons of flowers to obtain a litre of essential oil. Thus, pure organic and wild crafted essential oils can be very expensive and of course very effective.

## IMPORTANCE OF DILUTION:

In theory and in clinical practice, some essential oils can be used on the skin undiluted. However the safest application is via dilution with a carrier oil. So, when making your own preparations, you will need to dilute your essential oils accordingly. This means that you mix the concentrated essential oils with a fatty vegetable carrier oil like coconut, avocado, olive, sweet almond or jojoba. Trust me, 99% of the time, you will not want to apply them straight (i.e., undiluted) on your skin. This can cause "contact dermatitis" which is a pre-allergenic response that can prevent future use.

## Internal Use

Finally, and most controversially, some essential oils are safe for ingestion. The most basic form of ingestion is in culinary use where 2-3 drops are mixed in the dish. Another common internal preparation is to combine it into a drink. Remember that oil and water do not mix, so simply adding a drop to water will leave that drop undiluted. Some oils are irritants and all oils are very strong, so it's best to be safe and dilute it into some oil such as avocado or coconut oil first.

---
**CHAPTER 9**
---

# The Psychological and Spiritual Dimension of Healing

*"Once you have this inner peace between you and God, you can fight anything. Cancer is nothing"* – Dr. Raymond Yuen, MD

**T**raditional systems of healing have long acknowledged the effect of the mind and emotions in both health and disease. Traditional Chinese medicine links emotional and mental states to each of the bodys' organs. *(1)*

- Joy, laughter, talkativeness/speech and anxiety all correspond to the brain, heart and small intestines.
- Fear or fright correspond to the adrenals, kidneys, bladder and reproductive organs
- Sadness, depression and grief correspond to the lungs and colon.
- Worry and indecisiveness correspond to the stomach, spleen and pancreas.
- Anger and resentment or excitement corresponds to the liver and gallbladder.

Emotional qualities are not in themselves pathological, and all of them appear in healthy individuals. It is only when an emotion is either excessive or insufficient over a long period of time, or when it arises very suddenly with great force that it generates imbalance and illness. And the reverse is also true. Internal disharmony within the body organs can generate unbalanced emotional states.

Although ill health is usually the end result of the culmination of a number of disease causing factors, emotions such as fear, anxiety, frustration or anger can also bring on sickness. Think about this example of how emotions can affect their corresponding organs; if a child gets really scared, he or she can literally wet themselves. That's what happens when they have fear. Fear affects their kidneys and bladder causing loss of control of those organs.

So if you are stuck in the emotion of fear for a long period, organs that are going to be affected include the kidneys, bladder, adrenal glands and reproductive organs.

Grief and long-term sadness or depressions affect the lungs and colon. For someone stuck in these negative emotions as a result of, for example; the lost of a loved one (such as a spouse or child), or if they have been through a divorce, or have had a really emotionally trying time, this state of being really suppresses the immune system, which directly relates to the lungs and colon.

Worry affects the stomach, the spleen, and the pancreas. So, if somebody has cancer in any of these organs, oftentimes it's brought on by worry.

Diseases or conditions, which affect the heart, the small intestines, or the nervous system including the brain, may have their origin in the unbalanced emotional states of anxiety and nervousness.

Anger and resentment, or unforgiveness will affect the liver and gallbladder, which is your main detoxification organ. These emotionswill also have a negative impact on the lymphatic system that transports waste from the cells.

Now, before you go blaming your emotions and behaviour as the cause of your cancer, please remember that these correspondences between particular emotions and their associated organs, although useful to both the physician and patient are not meant to be mechanically applied or rigidly adhered to. Chinese medicine does not see them as precisely defined causes, but accepts them as yet another source of information with which to weave patterns of disharmony.

# PSYCHONEUROIMMUNOLOGY

In more recent times, a specific branch of medicine, Psychoneuroimmunology has been developed, which deals with the influence of emotional states on immune function, especially in relation to the onset and progression of disease. The basic premise of Psychoneuroimmunology is based on the concept that the mind and body are inseparable. It follows that stress and negative emotional states trigger the release of certain glandular secretions that compromise the immune system affecting the body's ability to resist disease.

Dr. Edward Bach, the originator of the Bach flower remedies knew of this connection between negative emotional states and disease when in the early 1930's he wrote: "behind all disease lie our fears, our anxieties, our greed and our likes and dislikes." (2) He made this revolutionary statement upon personal observation of his many patients, whose physical ailments seemed to be predisposed by negative psychological or emotional states such as fear, anxiety, worries, jealousy, poor self-image, anger and resentment. He believed that for true healing to occur, these negative emotional states must be resolved. "Treat people for their emotional unhappiness, allow them to be happy and they will become well," he states.

To use an analogy; just like the rust, which comes from iron that can corrode and destroy the same iron, so too can human minds damage the body. If we have learnt how to master our emotions, thereby producing positive thoughts, then our bodies will become stronger and healthier. If our minds produce negative thoughts, then like the rust on the iron, this will inevitably be a danger to us.

So, the old and familiar adage that, "A healthy mind is a healthy body," is especially relevant to cancer sufferers determined to beat this dreaded disease. When we are suffering from ill health, we need to also look in other directions besides just the physical. So, as well as feeding our bodies with a wide variety of cancer-fighting nutrients, we must also nourish our mind and soul with therapy such as meditation, prayer, uplifting music, laughter, compassion, physical activity, and so on.

The healing process is greatly enhanced when people are prepared to review and change, where appropriate, beliefs, attitudes and lifestyle factors. Previous stress patterns whether physical, mental or emotional, need to be addressed, or else treatments will only be acting as a "prop" and when stopped, the system will usually regress. So, we need to look at our attitudes with our jobs, with our family and with the ups and downs of life. These attitudes can either build or destroy. It's ironic that one of the few things in life over which we have full control is our attitude towards what life throws at us and yet most of us live our entire lives believing we have no control whatsoever. It is our attitudes that determine our physical health. Those who live in constant fear and worry of disease are the people who get it. If you are vindictive or malicious you produce tension in your body. When you feel hurt and rejected, there is tension in the body. When emotions such as hate or fear develop, they begin in the head first and then slowly seep into the body like poisons. To give someone a piece of your mind, you have to give up peace-of-mind.

Most of us blame people, situations and things "out there" for making us angry, sad or distressed. Yet it is not the outside things that cause us stress, but our inside perceptions that cause our emotional turmoil. Our perceptions and beliefs determine the way we react and respond to various situations; therefore, as we are willing to change our mental concepts around the situation, our emotional and physical responses change. Change the belief and the sensation changes. To help you get started on this new mode of thinking, read the axioms in the box below and make them part of who you are.

# Today is a good time to start:

| |
|---|
| • Today I will start with a smile and resolve to be agreeable. I will not criticise. I refuse to waste my valuable time. |
| • Today I refuse to spend time worrying about what might happen. I am going to spend my time making things happen. |
| • Today I will not imagine what I would do if things were different; they are not different. I will make success with what material I have. |
| • Today I am determined to do things I should do, and I firmly determine to stop doing the things I should not do. |
| • Today I will not indulge in self pity. Instead I will strive to be cheerful. I will take the time to appreciate and value the good things in life. |
| • Today I will act towards other people as though this might be my last day on earth. I will not wait for tomorrow. |

By applying these positive affirmations on a daily basis you will calm any inner turmoil you may be experiencing and in the process create a peaceful stress-free inner world by conscious intention alone.

The Mayo Clinic, a non-profit academic medical centre, based in Minnesota, U.S.A. lists the benefits of positive thinking: [3]

- Increase of life span
- Lowering of rates of depression
- Lowering of levels of distress
- Greater resistance to the common cold
- Better psychological and physical well-being
- Reduction in risk of death from cardiovascular disease
- Better coping skills during hardships and times of stress

# LAUGHTER IS YOUR BEST MEDICINE

*The arrival of one good clown exercises a more beneficial influence on the health of a town than the arrival of twenty asses laden with drugs.*
- SIR THOMAS SYDENHAM (17TH CENTURY)

Norman cousins wrote the book "Anatomy of an Illness"- Laughter is your Best Medicine". He was diagnosed with ankylosing spondylitis (a degenerative disease causing the breakdown of collagen), which left him in almost constant pain and motivated his doctor to say he would die within a few months. He disagreed and reasoned that if stress had somehow contributed to his illness, then positive emotions should help him feel better. He decided not to go down the drug route instead opting to use vitamin C, nutrition and laughter. He got a projector and all of the old comic movies of Buster Keaton, Harold Lloyd, and Laurel and Hardy. He watched 4 hours a day comedy and laughed with his friends. In less than a year his collagen disease was gone.

Well laughter is a good medicine. It releases chemicals that fortify the immune system. It helps in a thousand ways. So watch a comedy movie every day. Avoid watching cut'em up movies or movies that disturb the consciousness. Besides increasing energy and enhancing the immune system, laughter diminishes pain, reignites hope, enhances relationships, relieves tension, relaxes muscles and reduces the effects of stress. The greatest sign of mental health is to be able to laugh at oneself.

For this reason alone, begin setting a goal to make laughter a part of your daily life and to use humour in all your interactions with others. Some ways to facilitate this change are as follows:

- Begin by laughing at yourself.
- Make a joke at situations you would normally complain about.
- Watch children and use them as examples of how to laugh and take life lightly.
- Bring humour into conversations.
- Spend more time around funny people.
- Read funny jokes and share them with others.

- Watch funny TV shows and movies.
- Count your blessings while smiling.

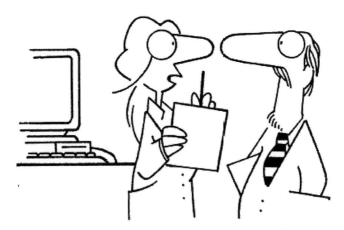

**"According to my research, laughter is the best medicine, giggling is good for mild infections, chuckling works for minor cuts and bruises, and snickering only makes things worse."**

## MEDITATIONS THAT ARE KNOWN TO HELP CANCER PATIENTS

Meditation will help in the cure of almost any type of disease because it involves activating your life force or vital energies. In general, meditation involves being able to "go within" in quietness to be absolutely silent. When we practice silence, free of all activity, motion or disturbance we access a stillness of mind that helps us to put all aspects of our lives into clearer perspective. The psychological and physical benefits of meditation, once it has been firmly established include a slowing down of the brain waves which makes us feel relaxed and can relieve muscular tension, as well as a slowing down of the pulse, a lowering of blood pressure and a boost to the immune system.

When practiced diligently, meditation will overtime help establish and develop a new set of beliefs until they become part of our subconscious mind.

Dr. Benson of the Harvard Medical School has researched and tested the effects of meditation on the health and body. In his book called "The Relaxation Response" (1975) he states that meditation can treat diseases such as cancer because it helps the patient to release tension, bring the willpower to fight and the consciousness of being in control of the life. He has found that depression, hopelessness, loneliness and despair, psychological conditions very prevalent in cancer patients, can be alleviated with meditation. The meditation that Dr Benson advocates to bring best results is one that uses breath control and the silent repetition of a mantra to bring peace and tranquillity.

In his book "Cancer and Natural Medicine" (1996) *(4)* John Boik mentions the Australian psychiatrist Ainslie Meares who found that the most effective form of healing meditation for cancer patients was intensive sessions of imageless meditation, meaning "emptiness meditation" or "meditation without thought." This was the type of meditation that got the best results when people were using meditation in conjunction with allopathic medicine to treat their cancer.

Meares found that meditation:
- reduced the anxiety, depression and pain of those with cancer,
- inhibited the growth of tumours in 10% of the cases he studied (spontaneous remissions came in at 10% mark due to meditation),
- improved the quality of life in 50% of the cases,
- produced significantly longer survival rates,
- facilitated death with dignity in 90% of the cases.

All these things were possible because in emptiness meditation you let go of your thoughts to realise some stage of mental emptiness (free of discriminative thought). The mental stillness or emptiness of this state will cause your "chi" or life force to rise, which is the natural vitality of your body, and so when your "Chi" rises it can cure all sorts of illnesses. That's how meditation can cure.

When you let go of a negative habit or thought that you've been clinging to for decades this too can finally free your chi so that it can rise and produce a "spontaneous cure", which researchers like LeShan and Schulze have noted. That's why people who get cancer, but also hate their careers; when they finally say "the heck with it" and chuck what they've hated, but forced themselves to continue doing for decades, they can often experience spontaneous remissions. Finally the natural chi flow of their body, which they have been artificially holding back for years, can assume its natural circulation, and with this return to normality comes their cure. People who let go of the burden of wrong habits experience the same sort of thing.

In other words, if you build an artificial cocoon around yourself from forced habits, and which in turn inhibits your vital energies and natural joy for life, then you are going to get sick. You might not get cancer, and you might not get sick tomorrow, but you're going to get sick. Meditation is one sure method that helps you get rid of those solidified energy cocoons you've created for yourself so as to restore a natural chi flow to your body.

Meares encouraged "Effortless stilling of the mind" and discouraged the sort of active visualisation and imagery methods proposed by psychologists today. So the route of "guided imagery" for cancer was not his top recommendation.

Meares found that those who got the best results with their cancer had three attributes in common:

- Their meditation was profound and prolonged (the patients he studied attended at least 20 sessions of intense meditation.)
- There was little or no conscious activity during meditation (that's emptiness meditation.)
- They carried meditation into their daily lives.

Another meditation technique for cancer and other diseases is to visualise that your body burns away or is burnt by light and you become light only. After a while, that light turns into emptiness. The longer you stay there in that state of unknowing, the easier it will be for your chi to rise and produce its wonders. That's how you dissolve away old habits that you want to get rid of. That's how you banish sickness and increase your longevity.

What these meditation methods have in common that the researcher Ainslie Meares found - that cultivating emptiness, which is "absence of discriminative thought", is the most powerful type of meditation for healing. It's more powerful than thought-filled meditation like positive thinking or guided imagery.

So now you know the main meditation route for healing, which is the same route for spiritual progress or the mundane goal of changing your habits and behaviour. You now also know why it works, so the most important thing to do is to put it into practice.

## AN EXERCISE IN SELF HEALING

Sit comfortably in a chair and close your eyes. Take three deep breaths, breathing in slowly to a count of 5. Hold for a few seconds and then gently breathe out fully.

Then become aware of your whole body, starting with the top of your head. Allow the attention to pass over the whole body from the top of the head all the way down to the soles of the feet, and observing any tensions held in the body, let them go.

Repeat the word "relax" slowly in your mind to help let go of any tensions that you become aware of.

In that awareness let the mind become free of any concern or preoccupation.

Each time other thoughts distract you, just let go of them and return to that inner awareness and come to rest within.

> ➢ Now be aware of your feet on the ground,
> ➢ The weight of your body on the chair,
> ➢ The texture of the clothes on your skin,
> ➢ The play of air on your face and hands.
> ➢ Now, place your awareness on the senses:
> ➢ Be aware of smell....

➢ Be aware of taste....

➢ Be aware of hearing; of sounds near and far. Allow sounds to be received and let them rise and fall without comment or judgement of any kind....

➢ With your body completely relaxed and the mind clear, simply rest in this great awareness for a few minutes.

# THE HEALING POWER OF PRAYER

*"It's been proven that prayer actually can help heal people. Not only praying for yourself, but praying for others."* – Dr. Homer Lim, MD

Christianity, Judaism, Islam, Buddhism, every religion believes in prayer for healing. Some call it prayer; some call it cleansing the mind. The words may vary, but in times of illness, all religions look towards their source of authority to help them in the healing process. Many people have been willing to testify that prayer alone and God's intervention is what saved them. Even the Bible records examples of the effectiveness of prayer and healing, in the book of Genesis 20:17, 18; Numbers 12: 13; and Acts 28: 8,9.

Much anecdotal evidence in support of prayer comes from individuals praying for a loved one (known as intercessory prayer) with whom they have a strong connection and to whom they send sincere heartfelt healing intentions.

To scientifically evaluate the effects of intercessory prayer on healing, San Francisco cardiologist Dr Randolph Byrd conducted an experiment in which he asked Born-again Christians to pray for 192 people hospitalized for heart problems, comparing them with 201 not targeted for prayer. No one knew which group they were in. At the conclusion of the study he reported in 1988 that those who were prayed for needed fewer drugs and less help breathing. (5) Byrd concluded that, "based on these data there seems to be an effect, and that effect was presumed to be beneficial" and that "intercessory prayer to the Judeo-Christian God has a beneficial therapeutic effect in patients admitted to a CCU."

This study led to a resurgence of scientific evaluation of the effects of prayer on healing. One such example comprised a meta-analysis of several studies related to distant intercessory healing that was published in the Annals of Internal Medicine in 2000. The authors analysed 23 trials of 2774 patients. Five of the trials were for prayers as the distant healing (intercessory) method, 11 were with non-contact touch, and 7 were other forms. Of these trials, 13 showed statistically significant beneficial treatment results, 9 showed no effect and 1 showed a negative result. *(6)*

The authors concluded that the methodological limitations of several studies make it difficult to draw definitive conclusions about the efficiency of distant healing. However, given that approximately 57% of trials showed a positive treatment effect, the evidence thus far merits further study.

Many of the studies done over the intervening years indicates that the devout have better mental health and adapt more quickly to health problems compared to those who are less religious. *(7)* This is borne out in a commentary by the Journal of the American Medical Association (JAMA) December 1998 issue. In it JAMA specifically referred to the following works:

- Duke University reports that people who attended religious services at least once a week and prayed or studied the Bible at least daily had consistently lower blood pressure than those who did so less frequently or not at all.
- Harold Koenig, M.D. from Duke reported that in his study of elderly patients suffering from depression as a result of being hospitalized for a physical illness, the more spiritual they were, the quicker they reached remission from depression.
- A study of 1,718 older adults in North Carolina indicated that elderly people who regularly attend church have healthier immune systems than those who don't.

- A fourth study found that patients aged 60 or older who attended church weekly or more often were significantly less likely to have been admitted to the hospital, had fewer acute hospital admissions, and spent fewer days in the hospital during the previous year than those who attended church less often.

No doubt these pious individuals may lead more wholesome lifestyles. Also, belonging to a network of like-minded spiritual friends will have a positive impact on their health and well-being. The quiet meditation and incantations of praying, or the comfort of being prayed for, appears to lower blood pressure, reduce stress hormones, slow the heart rate and have other potentially beneficial effects.

To date, there are over 300 studies that prove that there is a healing power in prayer. Even though there are studies that report no benefit of having people pray for the sick, to my mind the question of whether intercessory prayer works is irrelevant. To me, what matters in prayer is that the individual focuses intently on communication with God. The very intensity of prayer has an effect on the one who prays and can be equivalent to direct intervention and healing from above.

As it says in the book of James 5:16, *"confess your faults to one another and pray for one another that ye may be healed. The effectual fervent prayer of a righteous person availeth much."*

Fervent prayer means intense prayer, passionately praying for someone and not giving up until you get it. That's how you need to pray. I truly believe that turning to God is the best thing you can do to fight cancer because ultimately He's our source, He's our creator, He can heal you in an absolute instant.

In Matthew chapter 7 verses 7-12 this is what Jesus said: *"Ask, and it will be given to you. Seek, and you will find. Knock, and the door will be opened to you. For everyone who asks, receives, the one who seeks, finds. And to the one who knocks, the door will be opened."*

God loves you. He wants a relationship with you. He wants to restore you to real health. All you need do is to ask fervently and have faith.

*"But when you ask, you must believe and not doubt, because the one who doubts is like a wave of the sea, blown and tossed by the wind."* (James 1:6)


Dr. Winston Morrow tells a good story which, although not exclusively about cancer healing, will give the reader a vivid illustration of how powerful prayer healing can be:

"Since 1988, when God miraculously healed me from having to have my left arm amputated at the shoulder, I have prayed for all of my patients. I have seen new shoulders, confirmed by before and after x-rays, tumours the size of grapefruits disappear and so very many obvious spontaneous and instantaneous healings that I can only conclude that God supernaturally intervened."

In the case of my healing, I had a white cell count of 75,000, my arm was swollen to almost twice the size of my other arm, it was blue and green with obvious gangrene, and the pain was so intense that I could not bear it. After I was told, "we have to amputate your arm at the shoulder tomorrow morning, because the IV antibiotics are not working and your whole body is infected and your heart will literally turn to mush," I checked out of the hospital.

A patient of mine who told me that God would not let that happen, almost had to drag me into my own office, and began to pray and I was beginning to get upset at her audacity almost to the point of anger.... Suddenly, I felt 10,000 degrees of sweet heat start at the top of my head and fill my body.... Instantly, not 5 minutes or an hour, but instantly, I got a new arm, no swelling, no discoloration, no pain...

This event was the impetuous for my praying for all of my patients before treatment begins. I do it with them, asking God for wisdom, and asking his Holy Spirit to do those things that I cannot do as a man. Sometimes the anointing is so strong that it is obvious that the Spirit of God is present.

I thank Him constantly for hitting me over the head and waking up this Christian who didn't believe that God is in the healing business today. I thought that it had all stopped with the apostles." *(8)*

Now, after reading that heart warming story and to help you stay focused while in the throes of battling your "dis-ease", I've put together a collection of Bible verses for healing that will encourage, inspire and help you remain positive as you read and meditate on their meaning, and take ownership of God's promises contained in them. In the Bible you will find many others.

# Jesus Overcomes FEAR

### Psalm 27: 1-3

The Lord is my light and my salvation; whom shall I fear? The Lord is the defence of my life, whom shall I dread? When evildoers came upon me to devour my flesh, my adversaries and my enemies, they stumbled and fell. Though a host encamp against me, my heart will not fear, Though war arise against me, In spite of this I shall be confident.

### Joshua 1:9

Have I not commanded you? Be strong and courageous. Do not be afraid; do not be discouraged, for the Lord your God will be with you wherever you go.

### Deuteronomy 31:8

The Lord himself goes before you and will be with you, He will never leave you nor forsake you. Do not be afraid, do not be discouraged.

### Psalms 34:4

I sought the Lord and He answered me and delivered me from all my fears.

# Jesus Eliminates ANXIETY

**Psalm 94:19**

When my anxious inner thoughts become overwhelming, your comfort encourages me.

**Peter 5:6-7**

Humble yourselves, therefore, under God's mighty hand, that He may lift you up in due time. Cast all your anxiety on him because he cares for you.

**Jeremiah 29:11-13**

For I know the plans I have for you, declares the Lord, plans for the welfare and not for evil, to give you a future and a hope. Then you will call upon Me and come and pray to Me, and I will hear you. You will seek me and find me, when you seek me with all your heart.

# Jesus Resolves ANGER

**James 1:19**

Know this, my beloved brothers; let every person be quick to hear, slow to speak, slow to anger.

**Exodus 14:14**

The Lord will fight for you, and you have only to be silent.

**Zechariah 4:6**

Then he said to me, "This is the word of the Lord," to Zerubbabel saying, "Not by might nor by power, but by My Spirit," says the Lord of hosts.

# Jesus Heals GRIEF

**Psalm 34:18**

The Lord is close to the broken-hearted and saves those who are crushed in spirit.

**Matthew 5:4**

Blessed are those who mourn, for they will be comforted.

# WORRY - Turn to Jesus

**Matthew 6: 25-30**

"Therefore I tell you, do not worry about your life, what you will eat or drink, or about your body, what you will wear. Is not life more than food, and the body more than clothes? Look at the birds of the air, they do not sow or reap or store away in barns, and yet your heavenly Father feeds them. Are you not much more valuable than they? Can anyone of you by worrying, add a single hour to your life? And why do you worry about clothes? See how the flowers of the field grow. They do not labour or spin. Yet I tell you that not even Solomon in all his splendor was dressed like one of these. If that is how God clothes the grass of the field, which is here today and tomorrow is thrown into the fire, will He not much more clothe you - you of little faith?"

# HEALING SCRIPTURE VERSES:

- Lord, your discipline is good, for it leads to life and health. You restore my health and allow me to live. (Isaiah 38:16)

- But he was pierced for our transgressions, He was crushed for our iniquities; the punishment that brought us peace was on him, and by his wounds we are healed. (Isaiah 53:5)

- My son; be attentive to my words, incline your ear to my sayings. Let them not escape from your sight; Keep them within your heart. For they are life to those who find them, and healing to all their flesh. (Proverbs 4:20-22)

- He (Jesus) said to her; "Daughter your faith has healed you. Go in peace and be freed from your suffering." (Mark 5:34)

- Praise the Lord, my soul and forget not all his benefits - who forgives all your sins and heals all your diseases. (Psalms 103:2-3)

- Who himself bore our sins in his own body on the tree, that we, having died to sins, might live for righteousness by whose stripes you were healed. (1 Peter 2:24)

- Is anyone of you sick? He should call the elders of the church to pray over him and anoint him with oil in the name of the Lord. And the prayer offered in faith will make the sick person well; the Lord will raise him up. (James 5: 14-15)

Here is an interesting piece of information I stumbled upon in my search on prayer and healing, especially for cancer:

## ST PEREGRINE, THE PATRON SAINT OF CANCER.

Peregrine Laziosi was born in Forli, Italy in 1260. He is known as the patron saint of cancer patients. St. Peregrine lived from 1260 to 1345, ministering to the sick and poor of Italy.

At the age of 60 he developed a cancerous tumour on one leg and foot. It spread and become so severe the doctors decided to amputate his leg to try to save his life.

The night before the operation, Peregrine prayed before an image of the crucifixion. The next day, when the doctor arrived to perform the surgery he could find no signs of cancer. Peregrine was miraculously cured.

The news of Peregrine's healing rapidly spread throughout the church. Christians began to invoke his name and ask for his intercession for relief from their suffering and for cures for their diseases. For centuries, cancer patients and their loved ones have prayed to St. Peregrine, the patron saint of cancer patients. Here is the prayer to St. Peregrine:

## THE PRAYER TO ST. PEREGRINE:

O Great St. Peregrine, you have been called, "The Mighty", "The Wonder-worker", because of the numerous miracles which you have obtained from God for those who have had recourse to you.

For so many years, you bore in your own flesh this cancerous disease that destroys the very fibre of our being, and you had recourse to the source of all grace when the power of man could do no more.

You were favoured with the vision of Jesus coming down from His Cross to heal your affliction. Ask of God and Our Lady, the cure of the sick whom we entrust to you.

Aided in this way by your powerful intercession, we shall sing to God, now and for all eternity, a song of gratitude for His great goodness and mercy. Amen. (9)

## AND HERE ARE SOME MORE PRAYERS TO MEDITATE UPON:

## PRAYER FOR THE SICK

Dear Jesus Divine Physician and Healer of the sick,
We turn to You in this time of illness.

O dearest Comforter of the troubled
Alleviate our worry and sorrow with Your gentle Love
and grant us the grace and strength to accept this burden.

Dear God, we place our sick under Your care
and humbly ask that You restore Your servant to health again.

Above all, grant us the grace to acknowledge Your Holy will
And know that whatsoever You do, You do for the love of us.
Amen.

## A HEALING PRAYER

Lord, You invite all who are burdened to come to you.

Allow your healing hand to heal me.

Touch my soul with Your compassion for others.

Touch my heart with Your courage and infinite love for all.

Touch my mind with Your wisdom, that my mouth may always put claim Your praise. Teach me to reach out to You in my need, and help me to lead others to You by my example. Most loving heart of Jesus, bring me health in my body and spirit that I may serve You with all of my strength. Touch gently this life which You have created, now and forever. Amen.

## PRAYER IN TIME OF SICKNESS

Jesus, you suffered and died for us,
You understand suffering. Teach me to
understand my suffering as you do;
to bear it in union with You, to offer
it with you to atone for my sins, and
to bring Your grace to souls in need.
Calm my fears; increase my trust.
May I gladly accept Your Holy Will and
become more like You in trial. If it be
Your Will, restore me to health so that
I may work for Your Honour and Glory
and the salvation of all men. Amen

# THE HO'OPONOPONO PRAYER FOR HEALING

In Hawaiian culture it is believed that withholding forgiveness leads to disease and disharmony. With that in mind, an Hawaiian healer Morrnah Nalamaku Simeona (1913–1992) developed a simple technique called Ho'oponopono (translated "correction" in Hawaiian) or to "to make right again." It involves four simple steps periodically thought about or said out loud during the day:

**Step 1:** Repentance –SAY: "I'M SORRY"

**Step 2:** Ask Forgiveness – SAY: "PLEASE FORGIVE ME"

**Step 3:** Gratitude – SAY: "THANK YOU"

**Step 4:** Love – SAY: "I LOVE YOU"

They can be said in whatever order feels right to you, and either out loud or quietly within your mind. The power is in the "feeling" and in the willingness to forgive and love. Saying them out loud does yield an extra power to them though.

## How Does Ho'oponopono Healing Work

Ho'oponopono practice is about clearing away old emotional conflicts and belief patterns. It works on the premise that dis-ease within the body is brought about by the way negative beliefs and emotions are behaving in your body and mind. This runs as a similar viewpoint to the view that much dis-ease in the body is related to stress.

However, this model goes beyond just negative emotions and belief patterns as all old data is taken into account. Much of whom you are as a person is underpinned by the way you think on an unconscious level. That type of thinking rarely comes to the surface; it remains more or less hidden, unless you go digging for it. However over the years you have changing viewpoints and can acquire conflicting viewpoints and develop dichotomies. All of which creates undercurrents and conflicts that can lead to a crisis both within the mind and the body due to the way the two interact. It is by clearing and healing these various sets of viewpoints, beliefs, values and data that this type of healing works.

## So: Step 1: Repentance – "I'M SORRY"

Repenting, or turning away from harmful beliefs and behaviours, or anything that has caused you sorrow or grief, is the first step to healing. Start there and say you're sorry. That's the whole step: I'M SORRY. In essence you are realizing that you are responsible for the (issue) in your life and feel remorse that something in your consciousness has caused this.

## Step 2: Ask Forgiveness – "PLEASE FORGIVE ME"

Forgive yourself and your body for not measuring up to its original blueprint of pristine health. Don't worry about who you're asking. Just ask! PLEASE FORGIVE ME. Say it over and over. Mean it. Remember your remorse from step 1 as you ask to be forgiven.

## Step 3: Gratitude – "THANK YOU"

Say "THANK YOU" – again it doesn't really matter who or what you're thanking. Thank your body for all it does for you. Thank yourself for being the best you can be. Thank God. Thank the Universe. Thank whatever it was that just forgave you. Just keep saying THANK YOU.

## Step 4: Love – "I LOVE YOU"

Say "I LOVE YOU". Say it to your body, say it to God. Say I LOVE YOU to your challenges. Say it over and over. Mean it. Feel it. There is nothing as powerful as Love.

When you put all the steps together into a full statement, it may look like this – *"To whatever that is going on within me, that's causing me to experience my present health status... I'm sorry, please forgive me, I love you, thank you!"*

Doing this causes your body to release negative thoughts and emotions, and opens you up to complete healing.

## To Summarise:

Obviously, cancer is a serious health condition. But cancer is not your life; it is not the essence of who you are. Your sense of self should be that you are Spirit, made in God's image and likeness. Do not allow your mind to dwell on the notion that "I have cancer"; don't empower cancer in anyway! Know instead, that you are a child of God, though you may be presently challenged with a condition called cancer.

Take these simple yet effective steps: Close your eyes then breathe slowly letting the air go deep into your lungs before slowly exhaling. Do it often, because it introduces much needed oxygen into your body and helps relieve stress. Go within, pray, meditate, watch Christian TV, read the Bible and listen to uplifting music; hear things that edify as well as say things that encourage and uplift.

Finally, know deep inside that Gods comforting and healing Spirit is always with you... much like a fountain whose healing stream flows eternally.

*"....and lo, I am with you always, even unto the end of the world."* (Matthew 28:20)

---

**CHAPTER 10**

---

# Miscellaneous Health Factors
# And Treatments

*The most powerful alternative cancer therapies are those aimed at strengthening all levels of a person's being at the same time – at reducing the body's toxic burden while also enhancing its multifaceted self-healing capacities and bringing the individual back to homoeostatic balance and healthy expression. – John Byrne N.D.*

## DR. BUDWIG'S FLAXSEED OIL
## AND COTTAGE CHEESE DIET

A truly remarkable all natural cancer recovery approach is German biochemist Johanna Budwig's "flaxseed oil and cottage cheese diet". Otherwise known as the Budwig diet, it is an eating plan that was developed to treat cancer. The diet is named after its creator, Dr Johanna Budwig (1908-2003), a 7 times Nobel prize nominated biochemist and cancer researcher who theorized that a diet high in polyunsaturated fatty acids, when combined with sulphur-rich proteins would reoxygenate and energize cells to keep cancer from spreading.

Her formula of flaxseed oil, a highly unsaturated fatty acid, when combined with the sulphur-rich low-fat (2%) cottage cheese, caused a chemical reaction that actually made the flaxseed oil water soluble, allowing it to be easily absorbed into the cell. This re-established the healthy electrical circuit charge to the cell membranes so that it could "breathe" again. These two foods, when mixed thoroughly and consumed daily are known to help suppress cancer cells by fostering greater oxygen circulation at the cellular level; and as mentioned in previous chapters, Dr Otto Warburg believed that insufficient oxygen was the key reason that normal cells turned into cancer cells.

Dr. Budwig claimed that multiple daily servings of her mixture (ie, one tablespoon of flaxseed oil is blended with two tablespoons of low fat cottage cheese and 2 tablespoons of freshly ground flaxseeds) could both prevent and cure cancer. She also discovered this dietary measure wasn't just effective for cancer, but also in reversing heart disease, diabetes, skin diseases, arthritis, autoimmune diseases, hormone imbalances and neurological problems.

In essence what Dr. Budwig discovered was the important role that the essential fatty acids (omega-3 and 6) played in oxygenating cells. In her attempt to reverse cancer (an anaerobic condition) Dr. Budwig believed she needed to quickly replenish her patient's bodies with sufficient EFAs and flaxseed oil was the highest source around. The way that cottage cheese comes into play is the following; in researching how to most efficiently get the depleted essential fatty acids back into our bodies, Dr. Budwig found that the body's assimilation and use of essential fatty acids was greatly enhanced when the fatty acids were combined with sulphur-based proteins. Cottage cheese is one of the richest sources of sulphur based proteins and the most commonly used option around the world.

By combining flaxseed oil with the sulphur based proteins in cottage cheese the essential fatty acids bind to the sulphur based proteins and this makes them water-soluble and much more bioavailable to the body. Dr Budwig also discovered that there were certain vitamin and mineral co-factors that aided the body in its use of the essential fatty acids. The primary co-factors are vitamins B3 B6 and C and the minerals magnesium and zinc.

In addition to consuming the Budwig Diet of flaxseed and cottage cheese, Dr Budwig also recommended making other dietary and lifestyle change to help increase protection against cancer and other degenerative diseases. These dietary changes and restrictions are broadly along the lines as outlined in this book such as eliminating from your diet all processed foods and damaging hydrogenated fats and oils, and most importantly sugar, and consuming only wholesome foods, vegetable juices and herbal teas.

Dr Budwig reportedly accumulated over 1,000 documented cases of cancer recovery with her special dietary approach over a 50 year period. And although some people using this approach have reported a remarkably fast disappearance of tumours, sometimes in just a few months, others may take longer. Dr Budwig recommended that people with cancer or serious illness should stay on this protocol for 3 to 5 years to achieve true healing.

## BUDWIG DIET FLAXSEED OIL AND COTTAGE CHEESE RECIPE

The Budwig diet protocol consists of eating multiple daily servings of the Budwig Diet recipe in addition to increasing your intake of fruits, vegetables and fresh juices.

Generally, each tablespoon (15 ml) of flaxseed oil is blended with 2 tablespoons (30ml) of low-fat (2% or less) organic cottage cheese. Mix only the amount you are consuming at one time so it is mixed fresh each and every time to avoid it going rancid.

One example would be to mix 2 tablespoons (30 ml) of flaxseed oil with 4 tablespoons (60ml) of cottage cheese, consumed twice daily or more, depending on the severity of the health condition you are addressing.

The oil and the cottage cheese must be thoroughly blended at a low-speed using a handheld immersion electric blender for up to one minute, or until a creamy texture with no standing oil is achieved. Remember, you must blend only the flaxseed oil and cottage cheese and nothing else initially. And always use organic food products when possible.

Now once the flaxseed oil and cottage cheese are well mixed it can be supercharged by adding a tablespoon or two of freshly ground flaxseed to the mixture. Mix it in using a spoon. Do not buy pre ground flaxseed as flaxseed goes rancid 15 minutes after grinding. Instead, grind up the whole flaxseed with a small coffee grinder. Also, store the whole seeds in the refrigerator and grind fresh each time; either brown or golden whole flaxseed can be used.

For variety you can add other ingredients such as almonds, hazelnuts, walnuts, cashews, pine kernels, pecans, bananas, blueberries, strawberries, raspberries, cinnamon or lemon juice. It's usually best to place these extra ingredients on top of the completed mixture and enjoy as its own meal. The mixture should then be immediately consumed.*(1)*

**A word of caution:** Since flaxseed oil is highly unsaturated it readily oxidizes when exposed to air. If the oil becomes highly oxidized and rancid, it can be dangerous for cancer patients. It has a short shelf life and must be purchased as fresh as possible and always kept tightly sealed in the refrigerator. Never heat or cook cold-pressed (unrefined) flaxseed oil under any circumstances. If these guidelines are not followed, the resulting rancidity makes this oil unfit for human comsumption.

If you are suffering from cancer, Dr. Budwig recommended consuming 6-8 tablespoons of flaxseed oil (in the mixture) daily. Otherwise one tablespoon per day of flaxseed oil per 50kg of body weight can be taken to prevent cancer or as a maintenance dose to prevent reoccurrence. Whether you are being proactive with prevention or if you are on a healing journey, consider adding the Budwig diet receipe to your daily routine.

For a complete and detailed overview of the Budwig Protocol and other vital details of the overall diet, please visit the Budwig Institute oneline at http://budwigcenter.com *(1)*

# MEDICAL CANNABIS AND CBD OIL

Think cannabis and images of smoking pot or weed come to mind! But cannabis isn't just about getting 'high', it has been used in societies around the world for centuries as a remedy to treat a whole host of health problems such as pains to insomnia.

But in recent years cannabis and now CBD oil have received a significant amount of attention, particularly because of numerous online testimonials, claiming they can cure cancer and a number of other diseases as well. As a result the cannabis plant and its cannabinoid compounds have become the subject of numerous scientific and medical research studies over the past decade.

It is now well documented that this plant and its extracts can ease the side effects of chemotherapy and radiation such as nausea and weight loss. But new lab research shows that it may be effective in treating cancer itself. Researchers at the University Of Chicago Pritzker School Of Medicine have recently found that cannabinoid compounds (CBD) in cannabis have potent anticancer effects. (2) CBD stands for Cannabidiol. It's a phytochemical found in the hemp plant which is known scientifically as Cannabis. The researchers found that the cannabinoids stimulate apoptosis that causes cancer cell death.

## CBD Oil versus Medical Cannabis - What's the difference?

CBD oil is an extract from cannabis sativa (marijuana) and hemp (a plant from the cannabis family that's cultivated for its fibre and seeds). CBD oil is rich in cannabidiol, which is the major non-psychoactive compound of cannabis, meaning it doesn't make you high.

Medical cannabis (marijuana and marijuana extracts) contain the psychoactive compound tetrahydrocannabinol (THC). They will make you 'high' if you use enough, but it too has valuable medical benefits

# WHAT DOES THE SCIENCE SAY?

Researchers at St. Louis University Medical School discovered a signaling network hidden in the brain and throughout the entire body, named the Endocannabinoid System, or ECS. This network of receptors is specifically designed to use CBD, THC and other compounds in the cannabis plant. The cannabinoids interact with your body by way of these naturally occurring cannabinoid receptors embedded in cell membranes throughout your body. Both the therapeutic and psychoactive properties of cannabis occur when a cannabinoid compound activates these cannabinoid receptors.

So far, scientists have found more than 100 types of cannabinoids in the marijuana plant.[3] These natural compounds have different properties and chemical profiles and so far, only a few have been studied for their effects on cancer. In general, researchers have figured out that the cannabinoids fight cancer via at least two mechanisms that make it difficult for cancer to grow and spread. The cannabinoids are pro-apoptotic (meaning they trigger apoptosis, the process of natural cell death) in tumour cells while leaving healthy cells untouched. They also have anti-angiogenic properties (meaning they cut off a tumour's blood supply).

Another interesting way that CBD and THC compounds kill cancer cells is outlined in the CBD international website. [4] When these cannabinoid compounds connect to the CB1 or CB2 cannabinoid receptor sites on the cancer cell, they induce an increase in ceramide synthesis that leads to cell death. A normal cell does not produce ceramide when it is near CBD or THC, therefore it is not adversely affected by these cannabinoids.

The reason the cancer cell dies is not because of the cytotoxic (ceramide) chemicals, but because there is a small shift in the mitochondria. The purpose of the mitochondria within a cell is to produce energy (ATP) for the cell to use. As the ceramide is produced it turns up the sphingolipid rheostat. This production increases the mitochondrial membrane permeability to cytochrome C, which is a vital protein in energy synthesis. The cytochrome C is then pushed out of the mitochondria which ultimately kill the source of energy for that particular cell. Ceramide also disrupts the cancer cells digestive system that produces nutrients for cellular functions, and actively inhibits pro-survival pathways.

The key to the cancer killing process is the accumulation of ceramide in the tumour. This means that by taking therapeutic amounts of CBD and/or THC, at a steady rate over a period of time, the patient will keep metabolic pressure on these cancer cell death pathways.

Despite an absence of human clinical trials, abundant anecdotal reports that describe patients having remarkable responses to cannabis and CBD oil as an anticancer agent are circulating. Saying that, a number of recent laboratory and animal studies have reaffirmed the anticancer properties of various cannabinoids with promising results. For example;

- The International Journal of Oncology published a study in 2017 showing that cannabinoids successfully kill cancer cells in the lab, and it helps chemotherapy work better. *(5)*

- A review of 34 studies showed that cannabinoids kill glioma (brain cancer) tumours, but don't harm normal brain cells. *(6)* This is not surprising as CBD has incredible antioxidant potential as well. And for the brains delicate cells which are constantly under attack by free radicals, this is a very big deal.

- In animals, CBD has been shown to slow the spread of prostate and colon cancers. *(7)*

- A study published in 2018 found that a cannabinoid extract of hemp inhibits the growth of ovarian cancer cells. *(8)*

- A lab study showed that a cannabinoid compound called delta-9-THC kills liver cancer cells.*(9)* It also shows promise against lung cancer.

- CBD triggers apoptosis in breast cancer cells and it even stops the growth of aggressive and life-threatening breast cancer, especially the more difficult to treat triple-negative breast cancer. *(10)* It appears to interrupt the cells signalling abilities, thus preventing them from spreading.

- CBD is tripling the survival rate for pancreatic cancer, which is considered virtually untreatable. Although researchers from Queen Mary University in London have tested it only on laboratory mice, a similar effect in humans could be very possible, and could see CBD "in use in cancer clinics almost immediately," said lead researcher Marco Falasca. *(11)* The researchers think that CBD is a major breakthrough in cancer treatment, and especially for pancreatic cancer. It's one of the most aggressive types of cancer and has one of the lowest survival rates.

- CBD and THC also seem to supercharge the effectiveness of radiotherapy. They were both tested on a number of brain cancer cell lines that were also being irradiated - and the combination drastically slowed tumour growth when implanted into animal models. *(12)* In fact, the tumours started to shrink, say researchers of the study. Conventional medicine has few answers to brain cancer, which has a 5-year survival rate of just 10%, and so this discovery could be a major breakthrough, especially for those with advanced brain cancer.

Other researchers have shown that the cannabinoids in marijuana and hemp have therapeutic powers across a wide range of ailments such as;

- epilepsy
- Alzheimer's disease
- multiple sclerosis
- anxiety and depression
- chronic inflammatory diseases
- cardiovascular disease
- and more *(13)*

## THE BOTTOM LINE

- CBD oil has been studied for its potential role in treating many common health issues, including, anxiety, depression, epilepsy, pain, and more.

- Although CBD has been shown to help reduce symptoms related to cancer and cancer treatment, and even has cancer fighting properties, more research especially in the area of human clinical studies is needed to assess its efficacy and safety.

- Research on the potential health benefits of CBD oil is ongoing, so new therapeutic uses for this natural remedy are sure to be discovered.

- Though there is still much to be learnt about dosage and efficacy of CBD, results from recent studies suggest that CBD may provide a safe, powerful natural treatment for many health issues including cancer.

# Quality and Potency

More so than other herbs, quality can be an issue with certain CBD products, so it's important to seek out brands with a high degree of integrity that clearly disclose their sourcing practices and quality standards. Seek products that are completely organic, have a full spectrum of phytocannabinoids, which have been extracted by a method known as "Whole Hemp Low Temp Extraction". This whole hemp low temp extraction pulls out other hidden gems (terpenes, flavonoids and chlorophyll) in the hemp plant, which makes the solution clinically superior to using just isolated CBD. *(14)* Those of us in botanical medicine understand that the sum of all the parts of the plant is greater than any one single ingredient.

As for dosing, most of the literature demonstrates efficacy of CBD in the several hundred mg range, but that is for "single magic bullet" isolated CBD. Clinicians familiar with the use of CBD are reporting that efficacy can be achieved with much lower doses when using a full spectrum oil, some in the 10 to 25 mg CBD range.

As always, when starting new herbs and natural medicines like CBD oil, be sure to start slow, to understand how your body reacts and work up to higher dosages over time.

## THE ROLE OF PROBIOTICS IN CANCER CARE

Probiotics are live bacteria that are good for you. They live in your gut. They are best known for promoting digestive health. But probiotics have also been shown to improve mental health, skin conditions, immune function, reduce carcinogens in the gut and more. For instance, bacteria in the gut can decompose non-digestible plant matter into butyric acid, a potent anticancer agent.

You carry about 100 trillion bacteria in your gut whose weight is approximately 1 kg. You may be surprised to know that these bacteria outnumber your total body cell count by a ratio of 2:1. So you have twice as many bacteria as you have cells in your body! Under ideal conditions these 100 trillion bacteria live in a delicate balance of roughly 80:20 ratio of good bacteria to bad bacteria.

Certain bacteria such as lactobacilli and Bifidobacteria are beneficial "friendly" bacteria that support numerous vital physiological processes such as the manufacture of vitamin K, Biotin and other B-vitamins. These friendly bacteria also protect against the proliferation of "unfriendly" micro-organism such as infectious and putrefactive bacteria, fungi or yeasts like candida albicans and other pathogens.

Many of the bacteria in this mix are relatively harmless, unless we have compromised immune functions. Many bacterial infections are called "opportunistic" because they only happen when these unfriendly bacteria seize the opportunity while the host is weakened. These unfriendly bacteria can also produce metabolites that are carcinogenic and further a cancer process.

A healthy gut maintains a balance of the various intestinal flora, but with current lifestyles and the use of antibiotics, drugs, excessive alcohol and processed foods, this balance is often upset, and in someone dealing with cancer it can often result in a very lethal mixture of bacteria in the gut.

What happens in too many cancer patients is that the infection comes from the inside of the body, which is called "bacterial translocation", and not from outside. *(15)* Only one of three factors needs to be present for disease-causing bacteria from the intestines to slide through the intestinal wall and create a life-threatening infection in the blood (sepsis).

1. Disruption of the ecological balance of the normal intestinal microflora, resulting in over growth of harmful or pathogenic bacteria and fungi.
2. Impairment or damage to the cancer patients immune functions (i.e. chemotherapy and radiation.)
3. Physical disruption or injury to the gut mucosal barrier (i.e. surgery or drugs.)

Practitioners of natural medicine often recommend using probiotics, which means deliberately introducing "live" friendly bacteria into the intestines through food products (yoghurt, kefir, miso, sauerkraut) or through special supplements. The rationale for this is to control and minimise dangerous microorganisms by replenishing the intestines with friendly bacteria, whose functions also include detoxification, immune system support, micronutrient synthesis, hormone balancing and nutrition for the body's cells.

## What Probiotics Do to Cancer

- A study published in the International Journal of Cancer tested probiotics in 398 colon cancer patients who had surgery to remove at least two tumours. It found that probiotics prevented precancerous lesions from returning. *(16)*

- A study published in the proceedings of the National Academy of Sciences shows that probiotics may work as well as, or better than chemotherapy in treating liver cancer. *(17)*

- A 2017 study by Cleveland Clinic Researchers showed that probiotics reduce a woman's chances of getting breast cancer. *(18)* Dr. Stephen Grobmyer was one of the lead authors. He said the results show the potential to prevent cancer with probiotics.

- Probiotics can also ease some of the worst side effects of chemotherapy, especially nausea and loss of appetite. A 2009 study of breast cancer patients confirms that probiotics relieve chemo induced diarrhoea. *(19)*

## How to Take Probiotics

Probiotics include a wide assortment of favourable bacteria including lactobacillus, acidophilus and Bifidobacteria strains. Look for probiotic supplements that contain 5 or more strains of bacteria. Make sure the expiration date is at least a year away. The amount of good bacteria in probiotic supplements is measured in colony-forming units or CFU's. Look for brands with at least 10 billion. And a good probiotic formula also contains a prebiotic.

Prebiotics are the foods that these friendly bacteria eat in order to flourish. Fructooligosaccharides (FOS) is a prebiotic fibre that your body cannot digest but is a good food source for the friendly bacteria. Some probiotic brands include it as part of their formula. Both probiotics and prebiotics can also be taken in the form of fermented foods such as:

- Sauerkraut - this German stable is made from fermented cabbage and apart from having plenty of good bacteria it is rich in vitamins A, B, C and E.

- Kefir - it's a Turkish fermented milk drink, tastes nice and has a high concentration of probiotics. You'll find it in the refrigerated section of supermarkets, health food stores and Polish shops!

- Kombucha - is a fermented drink that feels like a soft drink because of its natural carbonation.

- Miso - is a traditional Japanese fermented food and a good source of vitamins B E and K.

## OTHER FACTORS IN BOWEL HEALTH

While a favorable balance of microorganisms in the gut is vital to the health of the digestive system, there are other factors, which are also vital to intestinal health. Ensure your diet is high in fresh fruits and vegetables as well as whole grains, which have good levels of dietary fibre. Include plenty of fluids, including filtered water. Cut out sugar, refined carbohydrates and other processed foods. Exercise and good stress management are also important for maintaining bowel health. Supplements such as vitamin A, Beta-carotene, zinc and the B complex vitamins also work to maintain a healthy digestive tract.

## EXERCISE FOR HEALTH

*"Eating alone will not keep a man well. He must also take exercise"* - Hippocrates 2,400 years ago

The benefits of exercise for the general population are well publicized. But what if you're a cancer patient? For years, doctors thought that cancer patients should rest to preserve their strength. That was completely wrong, according to Dr David Speakman. He is chief medical officer at the Peter MacCallum Cancer Centre in Melbourne, Australia. He claims that increasing evidence is showing that this outdated advice is actually causing cancer patients harm, as regular exercise can lead to a number of health improvements for cancer patients, including:

- Better aerobic fitness
- Increase muscular strength
- Improved quality of life
- Less fatigue [20]

*"Our attitudes to treating cancer have to change,"* Dr Speakman said. *"All cancer patients will benefit from an exercise prescription."*

He's not the only expert in this area to sing the praises of exercise – *"exercise has many of the same benefits for cancer survivors as it does for other adults,"* says Kerry Courneya PhD, Professor and Canada Research Chair in Physical Activity and Cancer at the University of Alberta in Canada. *"Some of these benefits include an increased level of fitness, greater muscle strength, leaner body mass, and less weight gain."* In other words, exercise for cancer patients can make them fitter, stronger and thinner- like anyone else who exercises.

The notion that exercise can help prevent cancer dates back to 1922 when two independent studies observed that cancer death declined among men who worked in physically demanding occupations. *(21, 22)* After these two early studies, the hypothesis of exercise having an anticancer effect languished until the 1980s and since then a paper in the Journal Medicine and Science in Sports and Exercise reported that more than 100 epidemiologic studies on the role of physical activity and cancer prevention have been published. *(23)* There's now abundant evidence that exercise can help prevent people from getting cancer. In this same paper which reviewed the 100 epidemiologic studies on physical activity and cancer prevention, it noted that:

"The data are clear in showing that physically active men and women have about a 30 to 40% reduction in the risk of developing colon cancer, compared with inactive persons. With regard to breast cancer, there is reasonably clear evidence that physically active women have about a 20 to 30% reduction in risk compared with inactive women. It also appears that 30 to 60 minutes of moderate to vigorous-intensity physical activity is needed to decrease the risk of breast cancer, and that there is likely a dose-response relation."*(23)*

More recent studies suggest that higher levels of physical activity are associated with a reduced risk of the cancer coming back, and a longer survival after a cancer diagnosis. A recent study reported from Sydney, Australia suggests that oncologists should prescribe exercise to all their cancer patients. *(24)* According to lead author Professor Prue Cormie of Australian Catholic University, *"people who exercise regularly experience fewer and less severe treatment side effects, cancer-related fatigue, mental distress, and better quality of life."*

*"If the effects of exercise could be encapsulated in a pill, it would be prescribed to every cancer patient worldwide and viewed as a major breakthrough in cancer treatment,"* Professor Cormie said. She now tells her patients to aim for 2½ hours of aerobic exercise a week, along with two to three strength workouts, such as weight lifting.

A study published in the British Medical Journal in the year 2000, which explored the reasons as to why exercise may be useful for cancer protection found that exercise affects several biological functions that may directly influence your cancer risk. These effects include changes in:

- Cardiovascular capacity
- Pulmonary Capacity
- Bowel motility
- Immune function
- Antioxidant defence
- Energy balance
- Hormone levels
- DNA repair [25]

## EXERCISE FOR CANCER PATIENTS: WHAT TO DO:

Every person's situation is different. Before starting a moderate to vigorous exercise program, see your therapist. The following types of exercise can help cancer patients, and everyone else, get back in shape:

- Flexibility exercises (stretching). Virtually everyone can do flexibility exercises. Stretching is important to keep moving, to maintain mobility. If you're not yet ready for more vigorous exercise, you should at least stay flexible.
- Aerobic exercise, such as brisk walking, jogging, and swimming. This kind of exercise burns calories and helps you lose weight. Aerobic exercise also builds cardiovascular fitness, which lowers the risk of heart attack, stroke and diabetes.

- Resistance training (lifting weights or isometric exercise), which builds muscle. Many people lose muscle, but gain fat, through cancer treatment. For those with a high fat-to-lean mass ratio, resistance training can be especially helpful.

Ideally, cancer survivors should do aerobic exercises and weight training as both types of exercise is critical to the overall health and wellbeing of cancer survivors. But whatever you do, don't get discouraged. Doing anything is better than doing nothing. *"The key is to start slowly and build your body's energy over time,"* says Professor Courneya. *"Your body has been through a lot and it is necessary to challenge it gradually."*

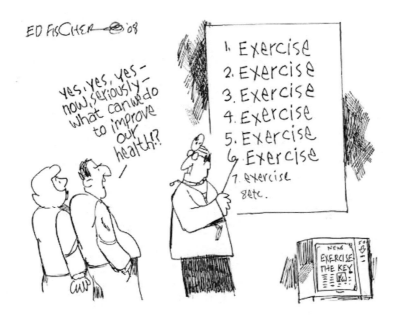

You can increase your physical activity without joining a gym, or even leaving the house. Just building more activity into your daily routine can get you started.

Here are a few suggestions:

- Take the stairs instead of riding the elevator
- Buy a pedometer (step counter) and increase your number of steps daily.
- Take frequent breaks throughout the day to stand, stretch, and take short walks.

Just remember, you didn't make it through cancer just to end up on the couch. Get together with your therapist or gym instructor, get an exercise program, and get moving!

# DETOXIFICATION IS VITAL

*"The main problem with today's oncologists is that they rarely consider the adverse effects of the toxins produced by the therapies they use. They wonder why their patients get sick and not well. It's because they're not dealing with the most critical aspect of therapy – detoxification."*

– Dr. Stephen B. Edelson

It would take a text book to explain about the dangers of personal pollution and the dire negative health effects of the environment we are living in. Suffice to say that toxins abound in our internal and external environment. In addition to our internal body toxins from gut bacteria and other metabolic processes, we consume and absorb many toxins from our external environment. These unavoidable toxins of modern life, in the water you drink, the air you breathe, and the food you eat, are building up in your body and destroying your health, increasing your risk of chronic and fatal diseases.

Research clearly proves that our bodies are not capable of eliminating all the different toxins and chemicals we inhale and ingest every day. They simply accumulate in our cells, (especially fat cells), tissues, blood, organs (such as colon, liver and brain) and remain stored for an indefinite length of time causing all kinds of health problems. Medical research has shown that the accumulation of these toxins leads to immune system dysfunction resulting in chronic ongoing inflammation, which results in fatigue, premature aging, degenerative conditions, cancer, etc etc. Our body is constantly endeavoring to detoxify itself, but if it becomes overloaded with toxins and impurities it will eventually malfunction and shut down.

Just how critical is it to get rid of toxins in your body? Well, Dr J.H. Tilden, author of "Toxaemia Explained" makes the admonition that "all sickness, all disease and all death is caused by the progressive accumulation of toxaemia (poison) in the body and the blood."[26]

Dr Sam Epstein (1926 - 2018), a professor of Occupational Health and Environmental Medicine at the University Of Illinois School Of Public Health, provides copious evidence that chemical pollution is one of the major causes for the soaring cancer rates.

Cancer patients who are undergoing conventional treatments are especially reliant on detoxification for survival. This is because, as the chemotherapy and radiation treatments kill large numbers of cancer cells, toxic debris is released, flooding the body and poisoning other cells and organs. That is why cancer treatments often result in extreme fatigue, sick feelings, foggy thinking and eventual collapse.

This is where natural treatments excels, as the right herbal and nutritional programs can help the body by stimulating healthy and gradual detoxification, resulting in these debilitating symptoms either dramatically decreasing or stopping all together.

So, if you are presently challenged with cancer, or want to prevent it, you must try to get rid of these cancer causing chemicals from your body. While your liver is

> **Phase 1 / Phase 2 Liver Detoxification**: is the natural two-step process the liver conducts to rid the body of toxins. During Phase 1, the liver converts toxic compounds into intermediate toxins. In Phase 2, the liver converts these intermediate toxins into substances that can be eliminated from the body, delivering them to the colon (via the gallbladder) or bladder for excretion.

the key organ in flushing toxins out, all cells, even brain cells contain detoxification systems whose effectiveness greatly depends on good nutrition. Magnesium, for instance, is involved in over 300 pathways, including the all-important phase 1 detox in the liver. Glutathione is another powerful antioxidant involved in both phase 1 and phase 2 detox pathways. But it gets used up everytime it deactivates a toxin molecule and we need to take phenomenal amounts. Unfortunately oral glutathione is poorly absorbed, however, I know of a product called "Glutathione Plus", which is a "reduced" Glutathione that has been clinically shown to increase blood Glutathione levels when taken orally. Another way to increase levels is to take the precursors that can help create Glutathione inside your cells: alpha-lipoic acid, N-acetyl cysteine (NAC) and s-adenosylmethionine (SAME). We also need Vitamins B3, B6, C, and E, Zinc, selenium, molybdenum and more. That's just to cope with the additional oxidative stress of our poisonous world. So you can see how important it is to have a diet, which provides adequate antioxidants along with other beneficial nutrients and where appropriate through nutritional supplementation.

## HOW TO PROPERLY DETOXIFY YOUR BODY

I wrote a book in 2015 called *"Getting Healthy Naturally"* where I explained in detail the measures you need to take to safely and effectively detoxify your body, starting with your gastrointestinal tract, then proceeding to your liver and kidneys with emphasis on blood cleaning nutrients, and also supporting organs such as the lungs and skin as well as the lymphatic system, to bring about a complete detox of the body.

Here's a quick review:

- First you cleanse your colon with specific herbs and nutrients to clean out all the toxic plaque and debris sticking to its walls. We call this the "remove phase" and its aim is to reduce inflammation of the gut mucosa.

- We then set about repairing the mucosal lining in the gut by supplying it with all the essential nutrients needed for the repair process. Some of these nutrients include omega-3 fatty acids, the amino acid L-glutamine, vitamins A, B9, B12 and the mineral zinc. We call this the "repair phase" and its aim is to help re-establish good digestive function once inflammation has been reduced by the clean out phase.

- We then need to replenish your gut with good bacteria (probiotics) that protect the flora balance, which in turn protects you as it's part of your immune system. We call this the "re-inoculate phase".

- While cleansing and repairing of the gut is ongoing, the liver can simultaneously be supported in its detoxification process by supplying it with a wide spectrum of nutrients, essential to the smooth operation of its phase 1 and phase 2 pathways. There are also many herbs and foods that also nourish, protect and cleanse the liver whilst supporting its detox pathways as well. Much of the dietary recommendations outlined in the food section of this book are strongly supportive of liver function. Some examples include all members of the brassica family as well as spinach, asparagus, beetroot, carrots, onions, garlic and avocados.

- With the bowel and liver cleansing and detoxifying more effectively, it's also important to assist and support other organs involved in drainage and elimination which include the kidneys, skin, lungs and the lymphatic system. After the liver converts toxins into water soluble compounds, they need to be eliminated by the kidneys. That means water is a vital component in this detoxification process and around eight glasses should be drunk every day, either warm or at room temperature.

- **Skin brushing** - the skin is responsible for eliminating many toxins. Simply brushing the skin with a dry brush can help to stimulate blood flow and lymphatic circulation, as well as remove dead skin cells.

- **Infrared Saunas** use radiant energy at a lower temperature to generate heat within the body. Radiant energy is able to penetrate more deeply into the skin and underlying layers, causing the body to sweat intensely and thus get rid of waste materials and toxins.

- **Foot Detox Spa** - this method involves simply placing your feet into a basin of salted water that contains ion generators. The ion generators are then supplied with very low electricity current that causes positive and negative ions to be produced, which then attract oppositely charged particles in the body. This process works by attracting charged toxic substances and then drawing them out of the feet into the water.

- **Chelation Therapy** - Chelation comes from the Greek word "chele". It means "Claw". It refers to the way an organic molecule can grab onto and bind to a metal. Chelation therapy is a very effective method of removing heavy metals such as mercury, aluminium, lead or arsenic safely from the body. For a gentle and effective heavy metal detox you could employ some of the following natural chelation methods:

  1. Vitamin C helps eliminate lead. Researchers have found that people with the highest level of vitamin C in the body also have the lowest level of lead in the blood. [27] Take at least 2000 mg daily. Liposomal forms are better absorbed.
  2. Coriander has been found to remove mercury, aluminium, and lead from both the body and the brain. All it takes is adding a decent quantity of coriander to your diet for 2 or 3 weeks. Try a handful of fresh coriander in a salad each day.
  3. Other powerful chelating substances to include in your diet are the seaweeds kelp and dulse which are excellent for removing mercury, especially from the brain; the green algae chlorella and spirulina, as well as apple pectin and malic acid, which are both found in apples and apple cider vinegar.

- Daily gentle exercise is fantastic as it helps get your heart rate up and flush toxins without putting too much stress on your body. It doesn't matter whether you walk, run, bike, swim or garden. Just elevating your heart rate twenty minutes a day will burn calories and send oxygen to your muscles and tissues.

## TO RECAP:

Pollution and toxicity are all around us and may cause a wide variety of health problems. Fortunately, we are born with an incredibly complex and efficient detoxification system to convert many of these substances into less damaging agents, which can then be eliminated from the body. This system for detoxification involves many different pathways, each dependent upon good nutrition to function properly. It starts with our own lifestyle such as adopting a good sound diet along with taking other positive steps to maximise our health status. The point to remember is that we are not helpless victims, trying to live our lives in an increasingly polluted world, but that we can exercise considerable control over our health. The recommendations in this section and throughout this book can help you achieve and maintain optimal health, even in the face of the many challenges before you.

# THE THERAPEUTIC EFFECTS OF MASSAGE

It is essential to involve the physical body and its musculo-skeletal system in the cancer-reversal process. Any therapist who's had the pleasure of watching a client's health and vitality improve through regular massage sessions would love to have everyone understand the benefits available to them from bodywork. Massage can help a person deeply relax, stimulate blood and lymphatic circulation, enhance the activity of the body's anticancer defences, and even release blocked emotions trapped in the body tissues.

Here are a few key points that should help you appreciate how regular massage can help you have a healthier life:

- **Massage helps to support your health** - Let's start with the fact that a full-body massage contributes to the proper function of your entire body. In attempting to remain healthy, your body's systems are performing functions constantly. The pressure and motion of the massage strokes assist in virtually all aspects of these functions. For instance, the nutrients that provide sustenance to the trillions of cells throughout your body — as well as the outgoing cellular waste — can be processed more efficiently with the aid of massage.

- **Massage reduces stress** - This one fact should inspire everyone to get massage regularly. People, who face a diagnosis of cancer, particularly for the first time, are often overwhelmed by a sense of anxiety and impending doom. This anxiety triggers the "fight or flight" response in the body, notably the release of adrenaline and leads to heightened muscular tension, elevated blood pressure, and other characteristic signs of being "under stress." Considering stress is responsible for most illness (not to mention those tense muscles), alleviating stress from your life can make a major difference in every aspect of your health and attitude.

- **Massage addresses the source of various health problems** - One of the tenets of natural healthcare is that, given the proper tools, your body will heal itself. Just think of how many of life's complaints are caused by an imbalance in your body — and massage helps to restore that state of balance. How do we know massage actually assists in this re-balancing act? Some of the functions measured during massage studies — changes in hormone levels, blood pressure, etc. — are regulated by your body. When these studies show an improvement in these functions, it offers measurable proof of the positive changes available through massage.

- **Massage at its core triggers reflex actions in the body to stimulate organs** – Massage can also help reduce swelling, correct posture, improve body motion, and facilitate the elimination of toxins from the body. Lymphatic Drainage massage, for example, can move metabolic waste through the body to promote a rapid recovery from illness or disease.

**However, A Word of Caution Though** – It is generally viewed that for cancer patients who have a toxic overloaded system, muscle massage should **never** be done until **after** the lymphatic system is working well; this would be **after** manual lymphatic drainage massage and/or dry skin brushing, plus the use of herbal lymph stimulators and other detox nutrients and compounds. It is important to emphasize that if lymph work is done **before** other immune-stimulating and cancer-fighting therapies are performed, lymph work theoretically might cause existing cancer to spread.

**Saying all that, a massage makes you feel better**, plus it's great to know more about how massage contributes to improved health. After all, we all want to be as healthy as possible. But there's something special about taking an hour or so out of your busy life just to feel relaxed and rejuvenated. Anyone who remembers how they felt at the end of a good massage session will tell you it's another great reason for making massage a regular part of your life.

## 3 "SUPERFOODS" – WHEATGRASS, CHLORELLA AND SPIRULINA

Wheatgrass, Chlorella and Spirulina are some of those things that fall into the "can't hurt" category when it comes to battling cancer. No matter what form of therapy you choose to undergo -- radiation, chemotherapy, surgery, or something more holistic – these 3 superfoods can only improve your results. If it were me, I would absolutely not undergo any radical therapy like radiation or chemotherapy. I would ingest large doses of these foods at every meal and pursue other anti-cancer strategies that have been proven far more effective, such as I have outlined in this book.

These 3 superfoods are so packed with healing properties that if pharmaceutical companies could patent them and sell them as drugs, they would cost €200 a gram and be front page news all over the world. Their ability to halt cancers would be heralded as a "medical breakthrough" and doctors everywhere would be urged to prescribe these substances to every one of their patients. It would be nothing less than a blockbuster, multi-billion dollar pharmaceutical achievement.

But they are not drugs and can't be manufactured in a drug lab, and so don't cost €200 a gram. In fact, they only cost on average 20 cents a gram and nature makes them for free.

# WHEATGRASS

If one single substance could claim the title of "superfood" the humble blade of bright green wheatgrass would be it. Hands down, if you want to detoxify, have more energy, stay alkalized and oxygenated, adding wheatgrass to your daily diet is a great place to start.

Wheatgrass juice or powder is derived from the fresh sprouted leaves of the **wheat** plant and so **does** not **contain gluten**, which **is** only found in the seed kernels of the **wheat** plant, not in its grasses. It is packed with over 100 nutrients, including selenium, vitamin D and dozens of others. Studies show it has more antioxidants than most vegetables.[28] It is high in many key vitamins such as A, C, E, K and assorted B vitamins, as well as key minerals such as calcium, magnesium, selenium, manganese and zinc. In fact 30 grams of wheatgrass juice is nutritionally equal to 1 Kg of vegetables.

Because of this collection of nutrients, wheatgrass has gained a reputation for being a "superfood". Studies have shown these nutrients working together may help provide support for chemotherapy — People who are currently undergoing chemotherapy have a chance of experiencing side effects, which may be managed by taking wheatgrass. In a 2007 study published in the journal Nutrition and Care, patients who drank wheatgrass juice while undergoing chemotherapy experienced lower blood toxicity levels compared to those who only had typical supportive therapy.[29]

Wheatgrass is also rich in chlorophyll, the green pigment found in plants that play a central role in photosynthesis. In this process plants absorb sunlight, carbon dioxide and water to allow them to grow.

Chlorophyll is very essential to all life, it helps plants purify the air and raise oxygen levels. I like to call it the "blood" of plants. What's interesting is that this pigment may also benefit your health, such as:

- Improving red blood cell function — Chlorophyll contains enzymes that help cleanse your blood and increase its ability to carry more oxygen.*(30)*
- Controlling inflammation — Consuming foods rich in chlorophyll may be an effective way to help manage inflammation better, according to one study.*(31)*
- Promoting a healthier colon — According to findings derived from a rodent study and published in The Journal of Nutrition, researchers suggested that chlorophyll may promote a cleaner colon by inhibiting the production of colonytes (pathogenic bacteria) and cytotoxicity induced by dietary heme.*(32)*
- Prevents the growth and spread of candida albicans, the fungus that causes candidiasis.*(33)*
- Has anti-inflammatory effects and suppresses NK-kB, which is a signalling molecule linked to tumour development.*(34)*
- Stimulates Phase-2 liver detoxification.*(35)*

Wheatgrass can be juiced and mixed into other juiced vegetables. To juice wheatgrass, cut at the base of the blade and insert the tips into the juicer. Alternatively, you can get a shot of wheatgrass at your local healthfood store or some farmers markets in your area.

**Wheatgrass powder** - You can also source the powder form at healthfood shops and pour a scoop of wheatgrass powder into your drinks or vegetable smoothies to get the nutrients if you don't have a juicer at home.

# CHLORELLA

Chlorella is a type of algae (microscopic plant) that grows in fresh water. The name is derived from the Greek "chloros" meaning green, and "ella" meaning small. It is interesting to note that chlorella contains the most chlorophyll of any plant.

Chlorella can be thought of as one of nature's superfoods, simply because of the amount of nutrients that it contains. In fact, it is thought that chlorella contains every nutrient needed by the body. Some of the things that can be found in chlorella include protein (chlorella is 58% protein), all of the B vitamins, vitamin C, vitamin E, beta-carotene, minerals including calcium, zinc, magnesium and potassium, trace minerals, omega-3 fatty acids, nucleic acids, and chlorophyll.

Looking at the nutrients it provides, a well-informed nutritionist can only stare in awe: these are many of the nutrients needed by every human body, in near-perfect ratios! It's almost as if Mother Nature herself reached down from the heavens and said, "Here's the perfect food for all human beings..." and gave us micro-algae. They're that impressive.

## HEALTH BENEFITS OF CHLORELLA

Chlorella has a whole host of benefits for the body. These include:

- **Detoxification** – the chlorophyll in chlorella is a powerful detoxifier, and detoxification is vital for the body to operate at its peak. Chlorella seems to be also particularly good at removing heavy metals such as mercury and lead from the body. It also strengthens the immune system response. It is the fibrous outer shell of chlorella that binds with heavy metals and pesticides. Chlorella is also one of the best foods for cleansing the body's elimination systems such as the bowel, liver, and blood.

- **Digestion** – because of the high chlorophyll content, chlorella can relieve constipation, improve foul smelling stools, and greatly improve or even eliminate chronic bad breath. Chlorella also contains digestive enzymes such as chlorophyllase and pepsin.

- **Cancer** – interferon is one of the body's best defences against cancer as it stimulates macrophages and tumour necrosis factor. Chlorella increases the body's interferon levels, thus stimulating the activity of macrophages and T-cells, which enhance the immune system. Chlorella also contains carotenoids, which have anticancer properties.

  Of the few key phytochemicals that have been identified in chlorella, their known anti-cancer properties are nothing less than astonishing. And yet, this micro-algae probably works on many levels to combat cancer, going far beyond the handful of phytochemicals that have been identified. Remember: chlorella contains hundreds or thousands of phytochemicals, and very few of those have been identified or clinically tested.

- **Alkalinity** – it is important for the body to maintain a correct pH, however, many people are too acidic due to factors such as a poor diet, junk foods and stressful lifestyles. Most diseases start in an acidic environment so alkalinising the body to the correct pH is very important. Chlorella can help to balance and maintain your body's pH levels.

# SPIRULINA

*"Spirulina's predigested protein provides building material soon after ingestion, without the energy-draining side effects of meat protein; its mucopolysaccharides relax and strengthen connective tissue while reducing the possibility of inflammation; its simple carbohydrates yield immediate yet sustained energy; its GLA fatty acids improve hormonal balance; and its protein-bonded vitamins and minerals, as found in all whole foods, assimilate better than the synthetic variety. Spirulina can*

*generally be considered an appropriate food for those who exercise vigorously, as evidenced by the many world-class athletes who use it."*

  **- Healing With Whole Foods by Paul Pitchford**


**Also:**

*Some micro-algae have very favourable nutritional profiles for cancer and immune therapies. Spirulina and chlorella provide cellular protection with exceptional amounts of beta carotene (provitamin A) and chlorophyll. Chlorella, the algae to emphasize in those with the greatest deficiency, stimulates immunity in the treatment of all degenerative diseases by means of the "Chlorella Growth Factor" (CGF). Spirulina is rich in phycocyanin, a pigment with anti-cancer properties. Spirulina is also the highest plant source of gamma-linolenic acid (GLA), a fatty acid which strengthens immunity and inhibits excessive cell division.*

  **- Healing With Whole Foods**


As you can see from the two quotes above, the nutritional and anti-cancer properties of both chlorella and spirulina are rather remarkable. Like chlorella, spirulina is a microscopic plant (algae) that grows in fresh water.


## WHAT SPIRULINA CONTAINS

Spirulina is a truly amazing food in that it is one of the most complete food sources to be found anywhere in the world. It contains the following:

- High levels of protein – in fact, it is higher in protein than meat is! (65% by weight)
- Amino acids - it contains eight of the essential amino acids required by the body as well as ten non essential amino acids, which are often not part of a vegetarian diet.
- High levels of beta carotene
- All the known B vitamins, including vitamin B12 which is almost never found in plants
- Gamma Linolenic Acid (GLA)

- Vitamin E
- Minerals: calcium, magnesium, iron, zinc, potassium and many more
- Antioxidants, including one called phycocyanin that is only found in spirulina
- Mucopolysaccharides
- Chlorophyll

In fact, spirulina contains over 100 nutrients! For instance, a teaspoon of spirulina has more antioxidant and anti-inflammatory power than ten servings of vegetables.

### In relation to cancer prevention:

- It has many anti-cancer properties and induces cancer cell death. *(36)*
- Can potentially prevent cancer development.*(37)*
- Reduces the expression of proteins that increase cellular proliferation. *(38)*
- Enhances the immune system.*(39)*

# HOW TO TAKE WHEATGRASS, CHLORELLA AND SPIRULINA

Let's talk about how much of these superfoods you should actually take. The following figures are based on an average 70kg adult. Adjust proportionally to your own body weight.

### Wheatgrass:

- **Disease-fighting dose:** 60 grams / day
- **Maintenance dose:** 30 grams / day
- **Upper limit:** Consuming high amounts of wheatgrass regularly can cause a healing crisis that can make you feel nauseous and suffer other health issues such as headaches dizziness, fatigue and rashes.

## Spirulina:

- **Disease-fighting dose:** 20 grams / day
- **Maintenance dose:** 10 grams / day
- **Upper limit:** there is no upper limit. You can eat spirulina like food.

    If you eat "too much," you will simply get full.

## Chlorella:

- **Disease-fighting dose:** 10 grams / day
- **Maintenance dose:** 5 grams / day
- **Upper limit:** there is no upper limit, but introduce chlorella into your diet gradually and monitor your stools. Since chlorella can result in mild diarrhoea in some people, introduce it slowly. (Your body will adapt over a period of a few weeks, allowing you to take more.)

In all, the anti-cancer properties of wheatgrass, chlorella and spirulina make these superfoods absolutely necessary dietary supplements for anyone battling cancer or who may be at risk for cancer.

# AVEMAR - A Medical Food that Fights Cancer

Avemar is a potent natural compound that has been studied in autoimmune patients, and in a wide array of cancer patients, including those with breast, colon and skin cancers. More than 100 papers published in prestigious journals have reviewed clinical and experimental results with this extract, and it's now a medically approved substance for cancer treatment in Europe. In Hungary, where the product was developed, the mortality rate of cancer stopped rising and began declining after its introduction and in the wake of its increasingly wide-spread use. After reviewing the data, I strongly recommend that anyone with cancer consider this treatment.

Avemar comes from a patented process that ferments wheat germ with bakers yeast. The result is a supplement that performs three vital functions in the body:

- Helps the body regulate metabolism and more efficiently create energy from the nutrients we eat.
- Boosts the body's immune system and helps create stronger T-cells and macrophages (the cells that eat invaders and cancer cells).
- Helps the immune system target cancer cells and eliminate them by shutting off their "cloaking mechanism" that tells the body not to kill cancer cells.

The most exciting effect of Avemar is that it decreases glucose uptake by cancer cells.

Not only does this force cells to normalize, triggering apoptosis and slowing tumour growth, it starts to re-regulate glucose metabolism. And that addresses a serious side effect of cancer, called cachexia. As I previously described, cachexia is the rapid weight loss and muscle wasting that happens to many cancer sufferers. Patients experience severe malnutrition, even if they are eating. But the cancer cells have disrupted the normal absorption of glucose and other nutrients by healthy cells.

Since Avemar re-establishes the normal pathway for glucose metabolism, it allows better absorption of glucose and other nutrients by healthy cells. For this effect alone, this product has been invaluable. Avemar gives patients their lives back. It greatly reduces fatigue and helps them to maintain their weight.

Unlike many other nutritional products, Avemar has been studied extensively in humans. This is key - and since Avemar has immune balancing and anti-inflammatory compounds, it may be a product that would make sense to include in a cancer prevention regimen, too.In Europe, Avemar is currently the only non-prescription product with an officially approved label available on the market specifically for cancer patients.

Avemar comes in powder packets that you mix with water or juice and drink. One packet a day is the recommended dosage for an average adult weight of 70 kg. For 90 kg body weight, up to two packets are recommended. Once you mix the powder into a solution, it should be consumed within 30 minutes. Avemar may affect the absorption of other nutrients or medications, so it should be taken at least two hours before or after other dietary supplements and prescription and non-prescription medications.

For more information, visit http://www.avemar.com

---

## CHAPTER 11

---

# Putting it all together

*The successful approach to reversing cancer and preventing its future recurrence is always multimodal. No single therapy, technique, or substance can prevail against the complexity of this disease – John Byrne N.D.*

**N**o disease is more vicious than cancer. It kills hundreds of thousands of people every year. And the deaths are often long, drawn out and painful. For decades, the gold standard of cancer treatment involved surgery to remove tumours, chemotherapy to poison them and radiation to burn them away. But all of those approaches destroy healthy tissues along with tumour cells, and knock down the body's natural immune defences, which can lead to the cancer spreading.

The bottom line is that if you want to stand a chance of beating cancer, you can't just rely on the conventional medical approach alone; you need to incorporate into your treatment regime a comprehensive approach that also includes a range of natural healing modalities along with lifestyle changes.

As emotionally devastating as a cancer diagnosis is, it's also an opportunity to change your diet and lifestyle for the better, improving not only your quality of life, but your long-term survival. Cancer being a life-threatening disease asks people to look at their own mortality and the "meaning of life" for them. For many, it is the start of exploring their spirituality and there are no set pathways. For everyone cancer insists on change.

Every cancer patient that survives has a strong will to live. This strong will to live makes one willing to change everything. No excuses! You have to be willing to change your bad habits, your diet, lifestyle, even attitudes you may cling to.

In Dr. Ruth Cilento's book, "Heal Cancer", Ruth lists from her experience the prerequisites for healing. These are:

- To have the desire, commitment and the goal to live.
- To have a strong belief in the group, the doctor, the therapist, or whoever is the advisor and mentor.
- To have faith in the treatment itself and an intelligent interest in how it is carried out.
- To have perseverance and determination.
- To have a commitment to do everything necessary to reach the goal, even if it involves some sacrifice of comfort.
- To have peace of mind and to release fear and anger. This encompasses a feeling of self-worth and faith in God. It is a realisation that we are all part of the universal energy source, light, or whatever your belief is.

So, if you or someone you love has cancer:

- Don't accept that you have a life sentence.
- Do not panic - get educated (read this book and others, over and over.)
- Know that cancer is not a death sentence.
- Develop a healing plan and commit to it.
- Healing is within you. You can heal yourself with the right tools, resources and the right mindset. Make a decision to live.
- Have an attitude of victory. You have to believe a cure is possible in order to be able to heal yourself.

- Explore where you are today - your emotions, thoughts and decisions define your destiny.

## THE KEY TO CURING CANCER SUCCESSFULLY

- Identify all the imbalances.
- Recognise the root causes of the disease.
- Treat the problem systematically.

Oncologists mostly treat cancer like it was a localised disease, independent of the rest of the body. They consider the tumour, wherever it may be located, to be the "cancer". But in essence, these tumours should be looked upon as a symptom of a deeper cause, much like smoke billowing from a chimney is a symptom (or indication) of a fire (cause). When treating a person who has cancer, it's important to focus less on the cancerous tumour (smoke) and more on the underlying causes (fire) that causes the tumour symptoms to arise.

Andrew Scholberg makes the same point in his book "German Cancer Breakthrough", when he says that *"cancer is a symptom of a systemic disease of the whole body, no matter where the tumour may appear."* He makes the point that a cancerous condition is akin to a swamp and that swatting mosquitoes isn't enough, it's necessary to drain the swamp. In other words it is not enough to focus only on the tumour, we must address the condition of the body that gave rise to the tumour manifesting in the first place, we must quench the fire or drain the swamp figuratively speaking.

# YOUR CANCER ACTION PLAN

*Given the right combination of therapy and prevention, far more people can survive cancer and live long, productive lives than conventional cancer experts would ever deem possible.*

You don't wake up one day and have cancer. Once you are diagnosed, you really have had cancer for 10 years. It means you have been sick for at least 10 years. Cancer cannot grow in a healthy body. Having cancer indicates that something is out of balance:

- One thing for sure is your immune system needs strengthening.
- In addition, your body chemistry needs to be made less acidic and more alkaline because cancer can only grow and spread in a highly acidic environment, whereas healthy cells do best in an alkaline environment.
- There is also an urgent need to improve oxygenation at the cellular level, because oxygen enhances healthy cells and suppresses cancer cells. Every cancer cell has damaged mitochondria and so, does not use oxygen; instead fermenting glucose for energy. This important discovery was made by Nobel Prize winning scientist Dr Otto Warburg in the 1930s.
- And the final piece of the jigsaw, nutrient optimisation is essential to beating cancer. Good nutrition can make a huge difference and so, is an essential component of everyone's comprehensive cancer treatment program. A well nourished cancer patient can better manage the disease and its therapies.

In order to treat cancer effectively, I've developed a 7-step program that addresses the root causes of this disease and if implemented fully, will arm you with the foundational tools to reactivate your self-healing mechanism and achieve optimal health.

They are:

1. Transform and change your diet.

2. Detoxify the body.

3. Rebuild and strengthen the immune system.

4. Optimise healing with nutritional supplements and herbal tonics.

5. Address emotional, psychological and spiritual aspects of cancer.

6. Employ natural therapies to assist healing. Examples include Infrared saunas, Lymphatic drainage massage, Magnetic field therapy, Rife frequencies, and Oxygen/ozone.

7. Maintenance: Maintain the changes achieved with the previous six steps.

Let's go through each step in more detail:

## STEP 1 - TRANSFORM AND CHANGE YOUR DIET

Conventional oncologists know very little about nutrition, and rarely make any dietary recommendations. Even worse, some oncologists tell patients there is no relationship between their diet and cancer. The truth is your diet can make all the difference between recovering or succumbing to this nasty disease.

If you've already read through this book you will realise that cancer prevention and treatment goes light years beyond

> **Eat Your Vegetables**
>
> Some vegetables are much more powerful than others in preventing and treating cancer. The best vegetables to prevent cancer include:
> - Broccoli (especially broccoli sprouts)
> - Brussels sprouts
> - Cabbage
> - Cauliflower
> - Celery
> - Spinach
> - Kale
> - Parsley

what your oncologist knows or is willing to share with you. And throughout this book we have established that nutrition is one of the most important elements of the game plan to beat cancer. Compelling evidence tells us that specific nutritional changes and appropriate supplementation can vigorously fight cancer, significantly improving your chances of long-term survival.

## FOODS TO EAT - AND NOT TO EAT:

Do not eat foods that feed cancer cells. Such foods include anything made of sugar or that can be easily converted to glucose (sugar). Examples include:

- White and brown sugar
- Refined grains and flour
- Breads, pasta, rice, cereals
- Jams, biscuits, cakes, etc
- Soft drinks, energy drinks, alcohol
- Starchy root vegetables like potatoes

Remember, sugar comes in many different guises, such as dextrose, maltodextrin, agave and high fructose corn syrup, so become sugar-wise and learn to read labels.

- Do not consume dairy products because they promote the growth of cancer. They do not cause cancer but there is a relationship in the level of insulin-like growth factors (which promote cancer growth) and the intake of dairy.
- Do not eat foods that make your body prone to getting cancer, or that encourages its growth. Such foods tend to be acid-forming and pro-inflammatory. They include: all processed foods, red meat and pork, dairy products, hydrogenated oils such as margarine, soy oil, corn oil, canola oil, as well as other polyunsaturated oils. Hydrogenated (trans) fats and oils surround the cell membrane and damage the cell wall. This

interferes with oxygen transfer into the cell, resulting in low intercellular oxygen thus making conditions ripe for cancer initiation. The best oils to have in your cuboardare extra virgin organic olive oil, coconut oil and avocado oil.

- Go Gluten Free - Lessening gluten in your diet will reduce inflammation, so weed out wheat, barley and rye. Instead use buckwheat, spelt, and sourdough. In both sprouted and sourdough grains, the gluten is less likely to cause problems because the gluten is predigested.

# FOODS TO EAT INCLUDE:

- Lots of green leafy vegetables such as spinach, kale, collard greens, cabbage, beet greens and watercress. They can be eaten raw, lightly steamed or blenderized. Leafy green vegetables are rich sources of cancer killing phytochemicals, vitamins and minerals and are alkalizing and oxygenating for the body.

- Cruciferous vegetables; examples include broccoli, brussel sprouts, cabbage, kale, and cauliflower, are all considered having protective effects for most cancers.

- Antioxidant-rich colourful fruits such as strawberries, raspberries, blackberries, blueberries, dark cherries, blackcurrant, and pomegranates. The natural sugars in these fruits do not feed cancer cells (unless cooked, i.e. jams), because at the molecular level their electrons have a "left" spin, whereas the processed sugars that cancer cells love, have a "right" spin to their electrons.

- Eat sprouted foods - Sprouting is germination and it releases more bioavailable nutrients as well as deactivating some dangerous phytochemical compounds. Alfalfa sprouts and sprouted black beans are highly recommended.

- Focus on fermented foods - Fermentation accentuates the positive and eliminates the negative. For example the German dish Sauerkraut is made from cabbage, yet it has four times the immune building properties than the cabbage it come from. Fermented foods are teeming with friendly bacteria that promote digestive health and a strong healthy immune system. Other fermented foods include kefir, natural yoghurt, pickles, kombucha and brine cured olives.

- Get your omega-3 fats from cold water fish. The best types are:
  - ➤ Sockeye (red) salmon
  - ➤ Wild Alaskan salmon
  - ➤ Sardines
  - ➤ Anchovies
  - ➤ Mackerel
  - ➤ Herring
  - ➤ Scallops

You can also take a high quality fish oil supplement (not capsules). Make sure that the fish oil says on the label that it contains both EPA and DHA which are healthy fatty acids that reduce inflammation and are anti-carcinogenic.

Plant sources of omega-3 fats include:
  - ➤ Flax seeds
  - ➤ Chia seeds
  - ➤ Walnuts
  - ➤ Hemp seeds

- Eat Seeds - this is where you get your omega-6 fats. Omega-6 fats are also essential for good health, however, stay away from processed omega-6 oils. Black sesame and black cumin are good seed choices. Soak for 8 hours prior to eating and consume only a dessert spoon a day. Two other good sources are sunflower seeds and pumpkin seeds.

- And don't forget your nuts. Eating nuts can help reduce your risk of cancer and other chronic diseases. They contain many beneficial nutrients including omega-3 and omega-6 fats. Some healthy examples include:
  - ➢ Walnuts
  - ➢ Pecans
  - ➢ Cashews
  - ➢ Macadamias
  - ➢ Brazil nuts
  - ➢ Almonds
  - ➢ Pistachios

- Include in your diet the following "super foods" that bolster your immune system, provide much needed vitamins and minerals, fiber, protein digestive enzymes and antioxidant compounds, which all help to create an alkaline-rich environment that combats cancer growth and metastasis. Examples include:
  - ➢ Wheat grass
  - ➢ Barley grass
  - ➢ Spirulina
  - ➢ Chlorella

- Drink green tea - There have been numerous studies confirming the cancer boosting power of green tea. It contains polyphenol compounds which have been shown to suppress the growth and reproduction of cancer cells. Matcha green tea is 10 times stronger than regular green tea. Drink two to three cups daily.

- Flaxseed oil and cottage cheese - is a combination that was discovered by Nobel Prize nominee Dr Johanna Budwig. These two foods when mixed thoroughly and consumed daily are known to help suppress cancer cells by fostering greater oxygen circulation at the cellular level, and as I've noted throughout this book, cancer cells are suppressed by oxygen. A suggested protocol is to thoroughly mix a tablespoon of flaxseed oil with half a cup of low-fat cottage cheese along with two dessert spoons of freshly ground flaxseed and consume it daily.

- Spice up your life - Many studies show that turmeric, ginger, onions and garlic protect your body against cancer. For instance, it has been shown that Kyolic aged garlic lowers the risk of stomach, colon and prostate cancers. Those who eat 85grams of garlic and onions daily are 40% less likely to develop stomach cancer as those who do not. Ginger has been shown to inhibit cancer growth and numerous studies touts' turmeric, the colourful component of Indian curry powder, as an excellent cancer fighter.

- Juicing and Blending are both great:

  ➤ These methods of food preparation are so effective because nutrients are released (that are otherwise locked up inside the cell walls) making the food easier to digest.

  ➤ Helps your body detox due to its antioxidants, enzymes and many other nutrients that are readily available.

  ➤ It is recommended by Integrative cancer experts that cancer patients should consume 10 or more servings of vegetables per day; vegetable juice could meet part of this goal.

## KETOGENIC DIET DEFEATS CANCER:

Cancer cells preferentially use sugar but can't use fat for fuel. Healthy cells can use sugar and fat. If you cut off sugar, cancer cells will die. As you probably know, the cells in your body use one of two types of fuel: they either burn glucose (sugar) or ketones (fat). But as I said earlier, Dr Otto Warburg discovered that cancer cells live almost entirely on glucose. They can't convert fat into energy in an efficient manner. So, by eating a diet that provides adequate fat and no refined carbohydrates or sugar, you feed your healthy cells while starving the cancerous ones!

This is why I recommend a ketogenic diet as it is one that all but completely eliminates carbohydrates, while at the same time increasing dietary fat. The diet works by lowering blood sugar (including insulin which feeds cancer cells) while at the same time stimulating the liver to make special high energy molecules called ketones that healthy cells can use to make energy (ATP) for cellular metabolism. As an added bonus, the ketones that the diet produces have a direct toxic effect on cancer cells.

Some health gurus say you should limit the amount of fat you consume. I don't place any restriction on the amount of healthy fats you should eat. But notice I said "healthy fats." Healthy fats include monounsaturated fats such as olive oil, coconut oil and avocado oil. They also include animal fats, so long as the animals are raised under organic conditions. This includes organic chicken, lamb and grass fed beef in small amounts. Other sources of healthy fats include eggs, butter, avocados, coconut, omega-3 rich fish and nuts and seeds.

## STEP 2 - DETOXIFY THE BODY

The state of your body, how it looks and feels, as well as how it functions depends to an enormous extent on how well it is nourished along with its ability to detoxify. When the body is not cleansed, it causes disease. The unavoidable toxins of modern life, in the air you breathe, the water you drink and the food you eat are building up in your body and destroying your health, increasing your risk of chronic and fatal diseases. Medical science has shown that the accumulation of these toxins lead to immune system dysfunction resulting in chronic inflammation, which promotes cancer development and growth.

By following all the guidelines in step one concerning dietary changes you'll be well on the right path to successful detoxification. Detoxification occurs through Breathing, Perspiration, Defecation, and Urination.

In my previous book, *"Getting Healthy Naturally"*, I outlined in detail the measures you can take to safely detoxify your body by addressing all your Detox Pathways including your colon, liver, kidneys, lungs, skin and lymphatics. These measures include:

- Select herbs and nutritionals to detox your bowel, liver, kidneys, lymphatics and blood.
- Gut and liver cleansing and repair programs. If you have less than two bowel movements per day you are at a greater risk for cancer.
- Drink six to eight glasses of purified water daily.
- Lymphatic Drainage Massage to stimulate the lymph's circulatory network to help relieve blockages, speed up the removal of metabolic wastes and reduce water retention in the body tissues. Fifteen minutes daily on a rebounder is also great for improving lymph drainage. Dry skin brushing in the morning before your shower stimulates blood and lymph circulation.
- Regular use of a Far Infrared Sauna is excellent to sweat out a lot of toxins stored in fat cells just beneath the skin. Seaweed Mud Wraps can achieve similar results.
- Oil pulling is where you swish a plant-based oil such as coconut oil, sunflower oil or sesame oil in your mouth for 20 minutes, upon rising first thing in the morning, and spitting it out afterwards. The premise is that this action pulls out bacteria and their toxic metabolities, as well as other pathogenic organisms.
- Exercise - regular exercise is the penultimate weapon in the quest to remain strong and healthy. It improves the capacity of the heart, circulation, lungs and lymphatic flow. *'If it were a pill people would pay a high amount of money for that pill'*. Exercise cannot be put aside; it needs to be part of your day.
- Juice fasts will also help reduce toxins. Going on a juice fast for 3 days gives your body a rest from digestion so it can concentrate on cleansing, killing cancer cells, and the repair of damaged organs and tissues. The best vegetable juices for cleansing include; cucumber, spinach, celery, carrot, beet, parsley, coriander, kale, onion, lemon, wheatgrass, chlorella and

spirulina.

- Reduce your exposure to electromagnetic pollution (EMF's). EMF is classified as a class two toxin by the World Health Organization, the same classification as DDT and the heavy metal lead. The number one EMF source of toxicity in the house is microwave ovens, throw them out!

  ➢ At night, turn off all electronics and wi-fi.
  ➢ Mobile phones heat up the brain and may destroy the protective blood-brain barrier. Also, don't carry mobile phones on your body when possible.

# STEP 3 - REBUILD AND STRENGTHEN THE IMMUNE SYSTEM

I tell all my cancer clients that if they want to beat cancer, they have to become the "healthiest person in their locality". Unfortunately, by the time someone has cancer, their overall health is seriously compromised. That's why we build it up with good Nutrition, Detoxification, and Immune-boosting nutrients.

Doctors have long known that the key to beating cancer is via immunity. In fact, hundreds of studies have indicated that people with poor immunity are not only more likely to die from their cancer; they are significantly more likely to develop it in the first place. It's well known that people who are on immune suppressing drugs are way more likely to get cancer.

The immune system defends the body by attacking and cleaning out cancer cells. When a cancer cell forms, it creates markers (antigens) on its surface membranes, which the immune system recognises as foreign, and immediately kicks into response mode to wipe out the threat. Even a strong immune system struggles with this task. Imagine if it's already weakened, the challenge to sweep out cancer cells is that much more difficult.

The immune system gets weakened and dysfunctional for a variety of reasons. They include:

- High levels of stress
- Existing illness or disease
- Poor diet
- Deficiency of micro-nutrients
- Accumulation of toxins in the body
- Physical inactivity
- Lack of sleep and relaxation

## WAYS TO STRENGTHEN YOUR IMMUNE SYSTEM

All of the aforementioned recommendations re: diet and detoxification in this chapter and throughout the book can help boost your immune system. That's one of the amazing benefits of taking an holistic approach to health and utilising many natural forms of medicine simultaneously. These treatments and methods work together to re-build the system overall.

For a healthy immune system, do not eat foods that impair your immune system's ability to destroy cancer cells. These include sugar, junk food, fast food, processed food, foods that contain trans fats as well as hydrogenated oils and polyunsaturated oils. Also, stay away from foods that contain sweeteners, chemical preservatives and additives. Instead:

- Eat a balanced diet high in fibre and complex carbohydrates (vegetables), healthy fats only, with moderate amounts of protein. Eat fresh, wholesome, unprocessed foods.
- Increase water intake to 6-8 glasses per day.
- Supplement the diet with recommended nutrients.
- Exercise regularly.
- De-stress! Enjoy plenty of rest and relaxation.

# Examples of Immune-boosting Foods, Nutrients and Herbs

- **Mushrooms.** There are a number of mushrooms known as 'medicinal mushrooms' which can help the body fight cancer and build the immune system. These mushrooms contain a number of valuable cancer-fighting and immune boosting compounds including, polysaccharides, such as lentinan, beta glucan, lectin and thioproline. These compounds attack cancer cells, prevent them from multiplying and boost immune activity, including stimulating the body's natural production of interferon. Some of the very best cancer fighting and immune boosting mushrooms include shitake, reishi, maitake and cordyceps.

- **Garlic,** as well as **onions, leeks and chives**, have immune-enhancing allium compounds that increase the immune cell activity, help break down cancer causing substances and block carcinogens from entering cells.

- **Probiotics.** These are good bacteria that inhibit the growth of bad bacteria in the gut, and promote those that aid digestion and promote a healthy immune response to infection.

- **Vitamin C** is perhaps the most common nutrient associated with immunity and studies have shown it to have some very powerful effects. Research indicates that vitamin C increases the activity of specific infection fighting and cancer fighting white blood cells.

- **Vitamin E** is an antioxidant and immune booster. It stimulates the production of B-cells that produce antibodies to destroy bacteria. It also has a direct cytotoxic effect on cancer cells.

- **Beta-Carotene** increases the number of infection-fighting cells, natural killer cells and T-cells, as well as being a powerful antioxidant.

- **Vitamin D**, also referred to as the "sunshine vitamin" promotes cancer cell death as well as giving a boost to your immune system. Try to get at least 15 minutes of sunshine a day on bare skin, as well as supplementing.

- **Zinc** maybe the most critical mineral for immunity. Low levels of zinc have been associated with low levels of natural killer cell activity, abnormally low antibody response and weaker immune response.

- **Aloe vera** contains vitamins, minerals, amino acids, enzymes and other ingredients that stimulate immune function.
- **Liquorice** works particularly well when the immune system is suppressed by stress.
- **Cat's claw** has antioxidant and anti-inflammatory properties and contains alkaloids that stimulate immune function.
- **Echinacea** and **Goldenseal** have been clinically shown to be of benefit in opportunistic bacterial infections, common in cancer patients. These herbs enhance the body's defence mechanism by stimulating white blood cell and macrophage activity. Macrophages are like little 'pack men' that roam around the body, engulfing and destroying cancer cells as well as bacterial, fungal and viral organisms.
- **Beta-glucan 1, 3 / 1, 6.** This is an extract of yeast cell walls. When highly purified, it can be safely used to stimulate cancer-fighting T-cells of the immune system.

**In conclusion**:

A well functioning immune system is your best guarantee of winning the war against cancer.

# STEP 4 - OPTIMIZE HEALING WITH NUTRITIONAL SUPPLEMENTS AND HERBAL MEDICATIONS

When it comes to nutrient supplementation your conventional trained oncologist who typically knows very little about nutrition tends to be downright hostile, believing that vitamins, minerals and herbs will interfere with conventional treatments like chemotherapy and radiation, or have no benefit. Nothing could be further from the truth. This is backed up by plenty of research showing that efficiently designed nutritional programs can enhance the effectiveness of conventional treatments, reduce complications associated with those treatments, and prevent secondary cancers.

Nutrient deficiencies, which are prevalent today due to poor diet and a host of other nutrient depleting factors, can contribute to an overall weakening of the body and its immune defences, making a person more vulnerable to cancer. While an accumulative lack of essential nutrients can contribute to illness, including cancer, the correct fortification of these missing nutrients can start reversing disease. This is why I recommend nutritional supplementation as a frontline approach in treating this insidious disease, most often combining several dozen substances in a complete nutritional package.

In a nutshell; nutrients can improve cancer outcome by:

- Inducing apoptosis (programmed cell death) in cancer cells
- Revert cancer cells back to normal healthy cells
- Help the body to wall off or encapsulate the tumour.
- Improve immune functions to recognise and destroy cancer cells.
- Reduce the toxicity of conventional treatments or make chemotherapy and radiation more selectively toxic to cancer cells.
- Nourish the patient and avoids malnutrition.

## NUTRIENT COMBINATION IS THE KEY

The human body is a very complex system in which no component works alone. Many people tend to consume whichever vitamin or mineral happens to be the latest rage. They might hear that vitamin D prevents skin cancer or vitamin E prevents breast cancer or selenium is the star of the anticancer minerals; and so they begin to devour high doses of their chosen nutrient everyday. But that defeats the purpose. Taking a vitamin or mineral by itself, especially in high doses could actually do harm - in fact, when it comes to cancer, doing so could hasten the growth and spread of the disease.

Countless studies have shown that taking vitamins and minerals together in appropriate doses; as opposed to separately; can powerfully inhibit cancer at all its stages. The reason is that vitamins and minerals interact to restore each other's cancer-fighting power. Now I'm not going to tell you that taking a specific supplement will simply cure your cancer because that's simply not true! Like I said earlier, cancer is a multifactorial disease needing a comprehensive treatment approach. But what supplements can do is give your body and its immune defences a big boost, and even better, send your survival odds skyrocketing! But this isn't something you should tackle on your own. Seek out the advice of an expert who can tailor a supplement program for your specific needs.

In general terms, everyone including cancer sufferers should take a good multivitamin and mineral supplement for the efficient maturation and functioning of all cells involved in immunity, which include the following:

- Vitamins - A, C, E, D, B-complex and betacarotene
- Minerals - zinc, chromium, selenium, magnesium, manganese and iodine
- Also co-enzyme Q10, omega-3 fatty acids and probiotics

## HERBAL MEDICINES AGAINST CANCER

*"Behold, I have given you every green plant, and it shall be food for you."* **Genesis 1:29**

Herbs have been used for thousands of years to treat all manner of disease including cancer. No single herb is a guaranteed cure for any type of cancer, but many are non-toxic boosters of immune function and detoxification pathways; and many have direct cytotoxic effects on cancer cells. This is backed up by an enormous body of scientific information and research in the field of herbal medicine. Indeed many cancer drugs have been modelled on, or derived from chemicals found in plants. Some examples include the chemotherapy drugs vincristine, vinblastine, paclitaxel, docetaxel and camptothecin.

In contrast, herbalists acknowledge the existence of these active compounds but insist that the other less active components of the plant also have biological activity and are essential in presenting the medicine in a form which is easily absorbed, utilised and eliminated by the human body. By using herbs in their unadulterated form, a profound transformation in health can be effected via a modified and more balanced pharmacological response **without** the toxic side-effects that isolated active ingredients produce.

The pharmacological research done on known anti-cancer herbs has elucidated the various mechanisms by which they fight cancer at its various stages of development. These anti-cancer herbs work by:

- Inhibiting cancer-activating enzymes
- Promote the production of protective enzymes
- Stimulate DNA repair mechanisms
- Supply powerful antioxidants
- Modulate the activity of specific hormones that promote cancer growth
- Stimulate immune functions
- Enhance detoxification pathways in the body
- Ameliorate the toxic side-effects of chemotherapy and radiotherapy

There are literally thousands of herbal medicines that have anti-cancer properties. The following list offers some of the better studied herbals:

- Turmeric
- Astragalus
- Cat's claw
- Cancer bush
- Green tea
- Blood root
- Ginkgo biloba
- St Mary's thistle

- Siberian and Panax ginseng
- Red clover
- Pau D'arco

These herbs along with countless others, all work in a different manner and when combined in various combinations can attack cancer in all its various stages of development, from the initiation phase through the promotion phase to the metastatic phase where the cancer grows and eventually spreads. And the wonderful thing about using herbal medicine is that it does not harm normal cells in the body. This of course is the most desirable outcome when treating cancer.

Seek out the advice of a suitably qualified therapist such as a naturopath or herbalist knowledgeable in the area of cancer treatments, who can help guide you towards which combination of herbs is best for your particular therapy and specific needs.

## STEP 5 - ADDRESS EMOTIONAL, PSYCHOLOGICAL AND SPIRITUAL ASPECTS OF CANCER

For individuals afflicted with cancer, the healing process is greatly enhanced when they are prepared to review and change, where appropriate, their diet, lifestyle factors, and equally important, when unbalanced, their mental and emotional states. Previous stress patterns, whether emotional, psychological or spiritual in nature need to be addressed, otherwise the treatments will only be acting as a 'prop' or 'crutch' and when stopped the system will usually regress.

It's probably no surprise to you that emotions like anxiety, depression and grief can put great stress on your body. And it's probably no surprise to you that ongoing stress can take its toll on your immune system leaving you vulnerable to cancer. In fact, various studies have verified that people who are not as content and satisfied with their lives as their peers, have ten times the death rate from all illnesses. It is also generally known in cancer circles that patients who felt depressed and helpless, and who didn't take an active role in fighting their cancer had poorer outcomes.

## There may even be such a thing as a *"cancer personality"*.

Dr. W Douglas Brodie, founder of the Reno Integrative Medical Centre in Nevada, USA observed through his extensive work with cancer patients that patients who tend to develop cancer have several traits in common. Here are Dr. Brodie's observations:

1. Being highly conscientious, caring, dutiful, responsible, hard-working, and usually of above intelligence.

2. Exhibits a strong tendency toward carrying other people's burdens and toward taking on extra obligations and often "worrying for others"; having a deep-seated need to make others happy.

3. Being a "people pleaser" with a great need for approval.

4. Harbours long-suppressed toxic emotions such as anger, resentment and/or hostility.

5. Reacts adversely to stress and often becomes unable to cope adequately with such stress.

6. Has an inability to resolve deep seated emotional problems/conflicts, usually beginning in childhood, often even being unaware of their presence.

Now please understand that I am in no way implying that if someone has cancer, it's their own fault. What I am saying is that if you have any of these emotions or tendencies, you need to address them and ultimately let go of them. So; you can start being more attentive to your own needs. Find ways to let go of negative emotions like fear, anxiety, anger, guilt, worry and unforgiveness. And find ways to lower the stress in your life.

The easiest way to do lower stress is to engage in stress reducing activities. These include exercise, yoga, meditation, prayer, listening to uplifting music or even watching funny movies. They all help. You also have to practice changing the way you react to stressful events After all; we can't always control what happens to us but we can always control how we react to whatever happens.

Maintaining mental peace and having a positive outlook are hugely important to cancer prevention and its treatment. Make "happy" your new normal. A big part of life and health is a good sense of humour. Indulge often in healthy pleasures. Discover your greater purpose. Develop your spiritual connection to God. This is the best thing you can do to fight cancer.... God can heal you.

## STEP 6 - EMPLOY THE FOLLOWING SUPPORT THERAPIES FOR REVERSING CANCER

The successful approach to reversing cancer and preventing any future recurrence of this dreaded disease is by always incorporating a multi-therapeutic approach. No single therapy or nutrient can prevail against the complexity of this disease. That is why I encourage my cancer clients to also avail of the following useful therapies that provide physical support to their bodies as it fights to overcome cancer.

## INFRARED SAUNA

One of the most essential components of any cancer-reversal programme is to detoxify the body down to the level of its cells, of a myriad of toxins, heavy metals, chemicals and pathogens; and open up clogged elimination channels to move them out of the body. One excellent way of achieving some of this detoxification is through sweating. We've long known that sweating is not just a way to cool the body; it also has a very cleansing and detoxifying effect too. Research studies have shown that toxic substances including pesticides, heavy metals and many other fat-stored toxins are eliminated from the body through sweat. So it stands to reason that we should encourage our bodies to sweat more and thereby reap the health benefits of this simple bodily process.

One way to induce sweating is by using a sauna. Research shows that infrared saunas are most effective at inducing a detoxifying sweat. As opposed to traditional steam saunas that operate in excess of 75 degrees centigrade, infrared saunas generate radiant energy via electromagnetic waves at a lower temperature of 60-65 degrees celsius. This makes for a more comfortable sauna experience. In addition, radiant energy is able to penetrate more deeply into the skin and underlying fat cells causing the body to sweat more profusely.

## Improves the Immune System

The sauna's deep heat raises your body temperature inducing an artificial fever. As it works to combat the "fever", your body's immune system is strengthened. Combined with the elimination of toxins and wastes produced by the intense sweating, your overall health and resistance to disease is increased.

## LYMPHATIC DRAINAGE MASSAGE

Few people actually die of cancer. Rather, they die of toxaemia, produced by an excessive buildup of toxins. This is where the lymph system comes into play. The lymphatic system may be likened to an efficient plumbing system. If the plumbing's clogged, the bathroom isn't much use. Likewise, the lymphatics have to be capable of flowing freely and filtering out the toxins, otherwise a congested lymph system can adversely affect the body as a whole.

**DID YOU KNOW?**

Lymphoedema is a complication that can occur when surgery includes a lymph node dissection, which means removing one or more lymph nodes (lymphadenectomy) – the network of glands by which cancer can spread. When the lymph fluid cannot properly drain, it can cause tissue swelling and infection. Women who undergo breast cancer surgery are the most likely to be affected, but this condition can occur after other types of cancer surgery as well.

Lymphoedema can occur shortly after surgery, or even years later. Prompt treatment is essential.

Unlike the circulatory system that has the heart to pump the blood around, the lymphatic system doesn't have its own pump. So the movement of lymph fluid is dependent upon muscle contraction, diaphragmatic breathing and body movement. As muscles tighten, lymph vessels are squeezed and lymph fluid is pushed along and filtered through the lymph nodes on its way back to the venous blood supply. As a result, it is not uncommon to develop a sluggish lymphatic flow through inactivity, not drinking enough water and consuming the wrong types of food. The consequences of a poorly functioning lymphatic system will be a build-up of toxic wastes within the body tissues that ultimately lead to ill health.

The pivotal point here is that when the lymph circulation is impeded, the entire body tends to become more toxic and oxygen deprived. One could state that the lymph system is the beginning and end of all disease. Once you get the lymph circulating freely again, this enhances recovery from any illness by reversing the slow poisoning your body has endured over many years.

## Lymphatic Drainage Massage

This is a very gentle massage technique that is designed to stimulate the lymph circulatory network in order to relieve blockages, speed up the removal of wastes and reduce water retention in the tissues. The technique involves the use of gentle rhythmic strokes and pumping movements where the skin is methodically stretched in the direction of the lymphatic flow to clear blockages manually pump the lymph fluid and stimulate the lymph nodes.

I see a lot of clients at my clinic who suffer from a congested lymphatic system, so I usually do a few sessions of lymphatic drainage massage on them, and especially those suffering from fluid retention and the more chronic type of swelling known as lymphoedema, where limbs can swell up to twice or three times their normal size. Cancer patients are more prone to lymphoedema as a consequence of receiving conventional treatments like surgery and radiation.

# DRY SKIN BRUSHING

Your skin is the largest organ in the body and is capable of eliminating over a pound of waste products through its sweat pores each day, which is why it is often referred to as "the third kidney". The multitude of tiny sweat glands acts like small kidneys, removing toxins and cleansing the blood of health-destroying poisons.

If the pores in your skin become clogged up and can't function properly, this will place extra strain on the kidneys due to the extra load of toxins. Skin that gets clogged up with toxins and dead cells cannot function properly in eliminating such toxins. An excellent way to rectify this problem is by a technique known as "dry skin brushing".

Dry skin brushing on a daily basis is in an extraordinary gentle yet powerful technique that will:

- Remove dead skin cells and unblock clogged pores allowing the skin to breathe easily.
- Increase blood flow to the skin thereby helping your body to discharge toxic wastes.
- Increase blood flow to the skin, allowing more nourishment and oxygen to reach the skin.
- Stimulate the peripheral lymphatics to drain away metabolic wastes and toxins that have collected in the interstitial spaces between body cells.
- Stimulate nerve endings that help rejuvenate the entire nervous system.

Daily skin brushing will quickly relieve puffiness and give your skin a smooth feel with a radiant look. It consists of spending approximately three minutes each morning just before you shower or bath, brushing your skin all over, using a natural fibre, long-handled brush. The technique is simple: you start at your feet and brush up your legs using long sweeping strokes. Next, brush your hands and up your arms. Then brush across your upper back and up the back of your torso. Brush your abdomen, neck and upper chest in the direction of your heart. The reason I'm giving you the specific directions to brush, is that you brush in the direction of the natural lymph flow only.

Do not brush your face as the brush is too rough for the delicate skin on your face, and also go gently on any other sensitive areas. Ideally, you should brush until your skin gets a warm glowing look, but do not brush so hard that your skin turns red and get scratched. After dry skin brushing, take a shower or bath to wash away any dead skin cells. I also recommend that you clean the brush in warm soapy water every two weeks and also, don't share brushes for hygiene reasons.

## MAGNETIC FIELD THERAPY

*"Electromagnetic Energy is the primary form of energy on which every living organism depends."*

The application of magnetic fields in the treatment of diseases is not a new idea. Magnetic fields have been applied since ancient times for all kinds of illnesses. In ancient China, magnetic field therapy was applied approximately 2,000 years before acupuncture was known. Hippocrates, Paracelsus and other famous healers of old, used magnetic fields to heal patients. In more modern times clinical evidence shows that cancers, subjected to a negative magnetic field, can start to reverse as the magnetic energy helps to restore oxygen levels and reduce acidity in the tissues.

Electromagnetic energy and the human body have an important inter-relationship. The human body produces subtle magnetic fields that are generated by chemical reactions within the cells and the weak electrical currents of the nervous system. Our bodies' function by way of these finely coordinated networks of electromagnetic fields that regulate most bodily functions and keeps them in their natural balance.

When the body's frequency patterns are disturbed, for example, through injury, excessive stress, lack of movement, or poor eating habits, it is often the start of a chain of effects that lead to poor quality of life or even illness. Magnetic field therapy helps to rebalance these frequency patterns, strengthening the body and its functions, thereby increasing both physical and emotional wellbeing.

The goal of magnetic field therapy is to give the diseased organ, through the application of magnetic fields, the ability to repair the functional and structural defects caused by the illness. The body gets stimulated to activate and strengthen its weakened physiological healing processes. The magnetic fields produced by magnets or electromagnetic generating devices are able to penetrate the human body and affect the functioning of the nervous system, organs and cells. These magnetic fields can stimulate metabolism and increase the amount of oxygen available to cells.

At my Health Centre I use an advanced magnetic field resonance system the MRS 2000+ which produces pulsating magnetic fields that match the frequency patterns of our daily biorhythms. Scientists learned that when magnetic fields are pulsed, their effect is considerably enhanced. It covers the innate vibration of a wider range of cells and tissues, optimising the energy potential of the cells, strengthening the body and its functions and increasing physical and emotional wellbeing.

## THE RIFE FREQUENCY GENERATOR

I covered in detail the history of this remarkable machine in chapter 1 and how it can literally shatter microbes that cause or contribute to the development of cancer. Dr Royal Raymond Rife discovered that if you play a resonant electromagnetic frequency to an organism (ie. bacteria or virus), the organism will oscillate or vibrate to the frequency until it bursts; much like the way an opera singer can shatter a crystal glass with the right singing note.

Rife's frequency generator was not designed to directly kill cancer cells, but only to kill the microbes inside the cancer cells causing the cancer, as well as similar microbes in the blood and in the spaces between cells. This phenomenon is medically referred to as **"electroporation"** and its killing disruption leads to the cancer cells malfunction and death. And the good news is that normal healthy cells that don't harbour these cancer microbes are unaffected by these lethal frequencies.

It is worth mentioning that although Rife found a microorganism to be a casual factor to cancer; this did not mean he was proving cancer to be an infectious disease. In fact, it is likely that the cancer-causing microbe Dr Rife identified is within each and every one of us. Rife agreed with and confirmed Bechamp's earlier theory of pleomorphism, that it is a body's inner environment which ultimately influences which form the pleomorphic cancer microbe would take. If a person's inner environment was healthy, then it would remain in itsharmless form. If, on the other hand, a person's inner environment was not healthy, it could devolve into one of the forms that might cause cancer.


At my Health Centre I use a **"Rife Medic-6 Quantum Radionics Resonator"**, which can produce a wide range of frequency signals to resonate the many pathogenic microorganisms in a person's body, such as viruses, bacteria, fungi, parasites, and other pleomorphic microbes, in order to shatter and destroy them.

The Rife Medic-6 Resonator can also be used to assist other functions in the body such as detoxing, speeding up healing processes, stimulating organs to function more effectively, and enhancing immune functions. A typical session on this machine involves holding a probe in each hand, connected to the Rife Generator while a pre-programmed treatment is selected from its display screen. Treatment times can vary from one hour to two hours.

# STEP 7 - MAINTENANCE - MAINTAIN CHANGES ACHIEVED WITH THE FIRST 6 STEPS

*"The unfortunate thing about this world is that good habits are so much easier to give up than bad ones."* – Somerset Maugham

The biggest reason people die after becoming a cancer survivor is they feel good, so they stop their treatments. Their cancer comes back and many of them die from it. Why is that?

It's because most of these people weren't actually cancer free. Instead their cancer was simply below the detectable level. This means they still had cancer. They just didn't know it. The cancer is just waiting for a chance to make a comeback.

So, how long should you be treating your cancer? The answer is simple: FOREVER. Never stop your natural treatments. They're a big part of the reason why you feel so good. By consistently following these previous six steps as thoroughly as possible on a daily basis is what's going to get you to your goal of being cancer free. Invariably however, because some people start feeling so good as their cancer starts regressing or disappears altogether, they may slowly start to slip fromtheir health maintenance programme, thinking that they no longer need to live by these six steps anymore, and they begin to revert to the choices that led to the illness in the first place. This misplaced thinking poses a real danger of the cancer returning.

These cancer-eradication protocols outlined in this book need to be made part of your new lifestyle rather than just used as a means to a desired end, and then to be discarded with. They are your new blueprint for living a disease-free life, but are only worth something if you choose to live by them. Thinking that you don't have to maintain your hard won health status after reversing your cancer diagnosis is like thinking that you only need to change the oil in your car once! Maintaining a vibrant state of health doesn't work like that, no more than exercising only once will give you a lifetime benefit - you have to keep working at it.

---

## CHAPTER 12

---

# A Practical Cancer Action Plan

***If you are too unwell to read much, then read this chapter first.***

*"I do not treat cancer so much as I treat patients who have cancer as a prime physical manifestation."* – John Byrne N.D.

**A**s I mentioned earlier in this book, I tell all my cancer clients that they have to become *"the healthiest person in their neighbourhood."* Becoming the healthiest person means three things:

1. Your immune system is strong enough to fight off pathogens that might attack (opportunistic infections) you while you're fighting cancer.
2. You have plenty of antioxidants that neutralize free radicals.
3. Your body is given optimum nutritional support to be able to cope with the physical and emotional stress of battling cancer.

If you're going to beat cancer, you can't afford to have anything but all three of these building blocks in place.

So in this chapter I'll offer some insights, regarding the "essentials" or "basics" of what you need to do right away to help reverse your cancer diagnosis. These suggestions will be helpful across several cancer types. Specifically, I'll recommend the best nutritional supplements, herbal medicines and others that effectively kill cancer cells, but do not harm the host and when combined synergistically, can be incredibly effective. Throughout this book I've shown that study after study indicates that supplements not only prevent and treat cancer, they can also ease the side-effects of chemo and radiation, and they can help patients recover faster after surgery.

You will be spared the onslaught of references in this chapter, though ample scientific documentation is found throughout this book to support the use of these dietary approaches and specific nutraceuticals as part of a comprehensive cancer treatment plan. It's no longer a question of whether supplements work, but which ones work best.

The following are supplements every cancer patient should consider taking:

# PROBIOTICS

You can eat all the best and most nourishing foods in the world but you will derive little or no benefit from them if you do not have the right balance of beneficial bacteria in your gut. Most significantly, your gut bacteria seem to get ill first - they lose their overall numbers and diversity, and you cannot get well until they get well. So, take a daily multi-strain probiotic that contains five or more different strains of bacteria. The amount of good bacteria in probiotic supplements is measured in colony-forming units or CFUs. Look for brands with at least 10 billion bacteria.

## MULTIVITAMIN / MINERAL COMPLEX

This is your insurance policy. Many nutrients are associated with cancer prevention. A good quality multivitamin / mineral supplement will help fill the nutrient gaps in your diet helping to offset problems associated with poor dietary choices. In addition, many of these nutrients have been shown to re-regulate the cancer cell, change the underlying cause of this disease and nourish the host to upregulate their cancer killing mechanisms.

# VITAMIN D

Vitamin D is a real cancer-fighting superstar. This vital vitamin can help cut your cancer risk and support your recovery after a diagnosis. Also known as the sunshine vitamin, it is produced by the body as a response to sun exposure. It can also be consumed in food or supplements.

## What it does to Cancer:

For decades, researchers knew that cancer rates were higher in people who lived further from the equator, where people get less sun and had lower vitamin D levels. But in recent years researchers have discovered that vitamin D can prevent and treat cancer. A large 2014 study of more than 17,000 cancer patients found that those who keep their vitamin D levels high have a better chance of surviving. They also remain in remission longer. But the benefits of vitamin D go much further. More than 60 studies have found that high levels of vitamin D are associated with a lower risk of up to 17 different types of cancer. This includes some of the most common - colon, breast, prostate, lung and ovarian, as well as leukaemia and myeloma.

Vitamin D's role in cancer prevention and treatment is just one of the reasons more and more doctors are starting to measure levels in everyone. So, if you are diagnosed with cancer, have your doctor check your vitamin D level. It's a simple blood test. If your reading is less than 20ng/ml, you need more vitamin D (ideal levels are 40-60ng/ml). Try to get 15-30 minutes of sun a day with your arms and legs exposed. If that's not possible, take a quality vitamin D3 supplement. I typically recommended 5,000 iu daily with food. You can also raise your levels by eating foods high in vitamin D3. The best sources are organic eggs, wild-caught salmon, and other oily fish such as sardines, herring and mackerel.

# VITAMIN C

Vitamin C is a powerful antioxidant and has many functions in the body's metabolism; many of them directly related to either preventing or recovering from cancer. There is a mass of solid evidence that this vitamin is essential for optimal functioning of the immune system. Among those immune components most actively involved in fighting cancer are the natural killer (NK) cells which are only active if they contain relatively large amounts of vitamin C. Vitamin C also boosts the body's production of interferon, which has anticancer activity.

Research also shows that vitamin C targets and destroys cancer stem cells. Cancer stem cells are what allow some cancers to come back after treatment. These stem cells are the seeds that propogate the growth and spread of new cancers. So, even if conventional treatment shrinks a tumour, unless cancer stem cells are wiped out there is a chance it can return.

Other research shows that vitamin C can repair genetic mutations that cause cancer; and that it can stop glycolysis in cancer cells. This is the process by which cancer uses glucose (sugar) to feed itself. By cutting off their food supply, cancer cells starve.

## How to take it:

Vitamin C is extremely safe, even in high doses. It can be given intravenously to help combat active cancers. Early trials show that patients getting IV vitamin C along with conventional chemotherapy did better than those getting chemo alone.

To take orally, I recommend you take a quality liposomal vitamin C supplement. The liposomal form is better absorbed by your body. Take 2,000mg a day.

# OMEGA-3 FATTY ACIDS

Omega-3 fatty acids are essential fats. That means your body can't make them. You must get them from food or supplements. Foods high in omega-3 include fish, cod liver oil, walnuts, flax seeds and acai berries. Omega-3 fatty acids form the building blocks of a number of anti-inflammatory compounds, thereby reducing inflammation, a major promoter of cancer initiation and spread. Studies show that omega-3 also prevents and fights cancer by turning on anticancer genes associated with the immune system and blocking tumour growth. A number of studies have shown that a high intake of omega-3 fats substantially lowers the risk of developing cancer, and of those patients diagnosed with cancer, when given high doses of omega-3's combined with chemotherapy led to a significant increase in survival. Other researchers have found that omega-3's are linked to tumour reduction in breast, brain and oral cancers.

Besides battling cancer itself, there's evidence that omega-3's also help cancer patients maintain their weight and not succumb to the wasting syndrome that is common in cancer patients known as cachexia.

Researchers have discovered that marine-based omega-3's are around eight times more effective at inhibiting tumour growth compared to plant sources of omega-3. Make sure that the marine-based omega-3 oil you take says on the label that it contains both EPA and DHA, which are healthy fatty acids. Follow label directions for dosage.

## CURCUMIN

Curcumin is a natural medicinal compound (flavonoid) extracted from the spice turmeric. It is the curcumin that gives the spice its bright yellow colour. Many quality studies provide strong evidence that curcumin fights a wide range of cancers. It is one of the most powerful anti-inflammatory substances found in nature, which means it inhibits compounds involved in the inflammatory response that can be involved in the initiation of cancer. In fact, unlike most anticancer drugs and supplements, curcumin has been shown to inhibit cancer at every stage - transformation, initiation, promotion, invasion, angiogenesis, and metastasis. The world renowned Mayo Clinic in Minnesota USA notes, "Laboratory and animal research suggests that curcumin may prevent cancer, slow the spread of cancer, make chemotherapy more effective and protect healthy cells from damage by radiation therapy."

## Dosage:

Cancer studies have used 2 to 8 grams of curcumin daily with varying success. In my own practice and as I've outlined in this book, I recommend a variety of herbs and supplements, which I know are far better than using just curcumin or any single supplement alone. Depending on the type and stage of cancer I typically suggest taking 1,000 - 3,000 mg daily of a well-absorbed form of curcumin.

# GLUTATHIONE

Glutathione is an antioxidant compound that needs to be present in adequate quantities within each individual cell for maximum health. It is found in fruits and vegetables and naturally produced in the body. It is critical to normal cell function including cell division and a healthy cell life cycle. In addition, it plays an important role in ridding the body of carcinogenic environmental toxins. It can also donate its electrons to other antioxidants such as vitamin C, vitamin E and lipoic acid so that these can be recycled and put back to work.

Many studies show that glutathione is lower in cancer patients and especially in those who are undergoing or have undergone conventional therapies such as chemotherapy, radiation and surgery. The importance of this is that without adequate glutathione, we have less ability to control free radical activity, which can lead to cell damage and many potential ill health effects.

When cancer patients are given glutathione, their overall health scores improve, meaning they suffer less serious side effects from conventional cancer treatments. A 2014 study published in the Eurpean Journal of Nutrition demonstrated that a special type of oral glutathione (setria) doubled the activity of natural killer (NK) white blood cells compared to a placebo. This is the form I use in my clinic and I typically recommend 500 to 1,000 mg daily on an empty stomach.

## COMBINE SUPPLEMENTS FOR THE BEST CANCER-FIGHTING IMPACT

Our bodies need many nutrients to fulfill the hundreds of biochemical reactions that keep us healthy. However, most of the studies mentioned in this book and elsewhere are testing only a single nutritional supplement or herb in isolation. This reductionist approach fails to consider the synergistic nature of nutrients. For example, consider colon cancer. It has been hard to pinpoint or show conclusively that nutrients reduce the risk. That doesn't mean they don't help. For example, vitamin D, folic acid, calcium and fish oil have all decreased cancer formation in the colon. Turmeric (curcumin) may also protect the colon. And evidence strongly suggests that a diet high in fibre could reduce your risk of colon cancer. So what would happen if a person had optimal amounts of all these substances? It only makes sense that it would help prevent colon cancer.

In my experience, taking multiple supplements and herbal elixirs to combat cancer and relieve its symptoms has a greater impact. Of course the best results occur when you combine supplements in conjunction with healthy diet and lifestyle changes as I've outlined in chapter 11.

## DIET AND LIFESTYLE CHANGES

Implement the following well-researched information as a starting point in your journey to conquering cancer.

- Change the environment in your body to make it a lot less acidic and more alkaline. Cancer thrives in an acid environment; and on the other hand your body functions best when its major fluids and most internal organs are slightly alkaline. Remember to drink enough pure water during the day.
- Eat fewer cooked foods and a lot more live, plant-based foods, especially a variety of deeply-coloured fruits and vegetables. In addition to excellent nutrition, they are high in fibre, rich in

enzymes that facilitate digestion, loaded with a wide range of cancer-fighting phytonutrients and insure a healthy acid/alkaline pH balance.

- Remember to consume foods each day that reduce inflammation, because inflammation adversely affects the immune system as well as the acid/alkaline balance in the body; - and inflammation is needed for cancers to flourish.

- Do things that cause more oxygen to be introduced into your body at the cellular level, because cancer cannot thrive where there is an abundance of oxygen. On the other hand, healthy cells thrive on oxygen, and deep breathing is one way to bring in more oxygen into the body, as is exercise. Also, eat raw green vegetables and drink their juices as they are rich in chlorophyll, and chlorophyll enhances oxygen circulation.

- Cleanse your body. Make a serious effort to detoxify, because it greatly enhances your body's ability to heal itself. You will find ways to help detoxification written in this book.

- Take steps to reduce stress. Meditation, prayer and moderate exercise are all very helpful.

# IN CLOSING:

## *What cancer cannot do:*

*"It cannot cripple love, or shatter hope, or corrode faith, or destroy peace, or kill friendships, or suppress memories, or silence courage, or invade the soul, or steal eternal life, or conquer the Spirit."* – Anonymous

Cancer is a nightmare. Don't leave it to fate. Make use of what we currently know. These steps and nutritional guidelines will not only help other health problems, they will give you your best fighting chance against cancer. It is time the medical community had a paradigm shift and stop thinking of cancer as some sort of localized disease, like a sprained ankle, and thinking that if we detect and destroy a tumour symptom early enough then the problem is solved. It is not enough to merely cut out or shink a tumour - we are dealing with a chronic metabolic disease that requires an holistic response, to include fundamental changes in our diet and lifestyle. While the bulk of this book is spent providing nutritional and nutraceutical facts to change the biochemistry of your body, my final parting comments are directed more at your soul, because cancer is a disease of the mind, body and spirit. Conversely healing involves healing physically, mentally and emotionally.

Today, our fast-paced modern lifestyles have taken us off the right track with nutrient-deficient and chemically-laden junk foods, a polluted environment, unhealthy lifestyle habits, and stress levels touching the Richter scale more times than naught. If this resonates with you, then isn't it time to slow down and start to experience some inner peace.

- Start your day with a smile and continue to give them away throughout the day with reckless abandonment.
- Refuse to spend time worrying about what might happen; instead spend your time manifesting what you'd like to happen.

- Take every opportunity to say: "I love you."
- Practice random acts of kindness.
- Think and act spontaneously rather than on fears based on past experiences.
- Savour and appreciate each day as though it might be your last, because the same holds true for all of us. You have the opportunity to be born again with a renewed vigour and purpose in life.

*From the bottom of my heart I wish you the very best on your Healing Journey back to Health and Happiness.*

*John Byrne*, N.D., B.H.Sc.

*Naturopath*

# References

## Chapter 1

1  https://www.tandfonline.com/doi/abs/10.3109/03014460.2013.807878

2  Vincent T DeVita, Jr.; Theodore S Lawrence; and Steven A Rosenberg, *DeVita, Hellman, and Rosenberg's Cancer: Principles & Practice of Oncology, 10th ed.* (Wolters Kluwer Health, 2016), 24.

3  https://www.cancer.org/cancer/cancer-causes/genetics/genes

4  https://www.davidrasnick.com/cancer/index.html

5  Hansemann, D. (1890) Virschows Arch. Pathol. Anat. 119, 299-326.

6  Boveri, T. (1914) Zur Frage der Entstehung Maligner Tumouren (Fischer, Jena).

7  Rasnick, D. and Duesberg, P.H. (1999) Biochemical Journal 340, 621-630

8  https://www.indiegogo.com/projects/what-cancer-really-is-books

9  https://drkelley.info/2013/09/14/dr-john-beard-and-the-the-unitarian-trophoblastic-theory/

10 https://www.dr-gonzalez.com/

11 Ewan Cameron & Linus Pauling, Cancer and Vitamin C, (Camino Books, 1979), p.4

12 https://www.ncbi.nlm.nih.gov/pubmed/8620425

13 https://med.stanford.edu/ludwigcenter/overview/theory.html

14 https://www.ncbi.nlm.nih.gov/pmc/articles/PMC3733496/

15 https://en.wikipedia.org/wiki/Otto_Heinrich_Warburg

16 Otto Warburg, Franz Wind, and Erwin Negelein. "The metabolism of tumours in the body," *The Journal of General Physiology,* 1927,8(6):519-530.

17 https://www.aqua-angels.com/wp-content/uploads/2017/04/Warburg

18 https://academic.oup.com/carcin/article/35/3/515/2463440

19 https://books.google.ie/books?id=rUCdBQAAQBAJ&pg=PA99&lpg=PA99&dq=william+russell+(1852-1940)&source=bl&ots=txlhbbez_d&sig=ACfU3U3_eJZRoRckqyOXWt8afq5nshJuFw&hl=en&sa=X&ved=2ahUKEwiq1LLHzqL

20   https://www.sanum.co.uk/gunther-enderlein/
21   https://ifnh.org/product-category/educational-materials/pioneers-of-nutrition/dr-antoine-bechamp/
22   https://www.cerbe.com/content/gaston-naessens
23   https://www.cancertutor.com/advanced_cancer_theory/
24   Bird, C. What Has Become of The Rife Microscope? NAJ43 (1984)
25   https://www.cancertutor.com/alt_critical/
26   Hess, D.J. CAN BACTERIA CAUSE CANCER?  New York University Press, 1997.
27   https://www.ncbi.nlm.nih.gov/pubmed/15944689?dopt=Abstract
28   Bach, E. The Twelve Healers:
     https://www.bachcentre.com/centre/download/healers.pdf
29   http://www.healingcancer.info/ebook/douglas-brodie
30   http://www.newmedicine.ca/bio.php

# Chapter 2

1   Morgan G, Ward R, Barton M. The contribution of cytotoxic chemotherapy to 5-year survival in adult malignancies. *Clin Oncol* (R Coll Radiol). 2004 Dec; 16(8):549-60.
2   https://usareally.com/1129-75-of-physicians-in-the-world-refuse-chemotherapy
3   Block, KI. Impact of antioxidant supplementation on chemotherapy efficacy: a systemic review of the evidence from randomized controlled trials. *Cancer Treat Rev* (2007),doi:10.1016/j.ctrv.2007.01.005
4   Morceau, F. et al. Biotechnol Adv 2015; 33: 785-97
5   Chen, X et al. Gene 2016; 592:86-98.
6   Zhuang W et al. Cancer Science 2012; 103: 684-90.
7   Bobilev I et al. Cancer Biol Ther 2011; 11: 317-29.
8   Ting HJ et al. Mol Carcinogenesis 2015; 54: 730-41.
9   Signorelli P et al. Nutr Cancer 2015; 67: 494-503.
10  Domokos M et al. Dig Dis Sci.2010; 55: 920-30.
11  Patel PN et al. Ann Surg Oncol. 2014; Suppl 4: S497-S504.

# Chapter 3

1 Pace, A. Journal Clinical Oncology, Vol 21, no. 5, p.927, March, 2003

2 Block, KI. Impact of antioxidant supplementation on chemotherapy efficacy: a systemic review of the evidence from randomized controlled trials. *Cancer Treat Rev* (2007),doi:10.1016/j.ctrv.2007.01.005

3 https://jamanetwork.com/journals/jamaoncology/fullarticle/2522371

4 Rothkopf, M, Fuel utilization in neoplastic disease: implications for the use of nutritional support in cancer patients, Nutrition, supp, 6:4:14-16S, 1990

5 Warburg, O., Science, vol, 123, no.3191, p.309, Feb. 1956

6 https://www.ncbi.nlm.nih.gov/pubmed/12442909

7 https://openheart.bmj.com/content/5/2/e000946

8 http://krispin.com/omega3.html

9 Holman, RT, Geometrical and Positional Fatty Acid Isomers, EA Emkin and HJ Dutton, eds, 1979, American Oil Chemists Society, Champaign, 283-302; Science Newsletter, Feb. 1956; Schantz, EJ, et al, J Dairy Sci, 1940, 23: 181-89.

10 Enig, Mary G. PhD, Trans Fatty Acids in the Food Supply : A Comprehensive Report covering 60 years of Research, 2nd Edition, Enig Associates, Inc., Silver Spring, MD 1995,; Watkins, BA et al, Br Pouli Sci, Dec 1991, 32 (5) : 1109-1119.

11 https://academic.oup.com/ajcn/article/79/6/935/4690254

# Chapter 4

1 https://nutritionandmetabolism.biomedcentral.com/articles/10.1186/1743-7075-8-75

2 https://www.ncbi.nlm.nih.gov/pmc/articles/PMC3614012/

3 Nebeling, L.C; et al. J Am Coll Nutr, 1995; 14: 202-208

4 Yale J. Biol Med, 2006 Dec; 79 (3-4); 123-130, Published online Oct 2007

5 Ruskin D.N. et al. Plos One 2009; 4: e8349

6 https://www.ncbi.nlm.nih.gov/pubmed/17694083

7   https://www.nature.com/articles/s41698-017-0024-2
8   https://babel.hathitrust.org/cgi/pt?id=hvd.32044020029617;view
    =1up;seq=18
9   Breuss, Rudolf with Hilde Hemmes. The Breuss Cancer Cure.
    Publishers: Walter Margreiter, Austria,  English Ed. 1997 by
    Australian School of Herbal Medicine.
10  Am Heart J. 2007 Jan; 153(1): 67-73.
11  https://www.ncbi.nlm.nih.gov/pmc/articles/PMC2815756/?tool=p
    ubmed

# Chapter 5

1   https://www.chrisbeatcancer.com/top-10-anti-cancer
2   https://www.chrisbeatcancer.com/wp-
    content/uploads/2013/01/Anti-Cancer-Vegetables-Study.pdf
3   https://www.chrisbeatcancer.com/the-giant-cancer-fighting-salad/
4   https://www.aicr.org/reduce-your-cancer-
    risk/diet/elements_phytochemicals
5   https://www.mskcc.org/cancer-care/integrative-
    medicine/herbs/diindolylmethane
6   https://www.academia.edu/7830474/Anticancer_effects_of_red_be
    et_pigments
7   Ferenczi, S. Treatment of Tumour With Beets; Preliminary Report.
    Zeitschrift fur die Gesamte Innere Medizin, v.10/22 (1955).
8   https://www.breastcancerconqueror.com/garlic-delivers-a-
    powerful-punch-against-cancer/
9   https://www.naturalnews.com/054316_garlic_antibiotic_properties
    _natural_remedies.html
10  https://draxe.com/7-raw-garlic-benefits-reversing-disease/
11  https://www.ncbi.nlm.nih.gov/pmc/articles/PMC6020439/
12  https://www.mskcc.org/cancer-care/integrative-
    medicine/herbs/lentinan
13  https://www.ncbi.nlm.nih.gov/pubmed/19048616
14  Cho, H. Et al; Food Funct 2015 6(5): 1675-83
15  Gonzalez-Sarrias, A. et al. Food Funct 2015, 6(5): 460-9
16  Seeram, N.Y et al, J Agrc Food Chem 2006;54 (25): 9329-39
17  Roy, S et al;  Free Radic Res 2002; 36 (9): 1023-31

18    Fuentealba, J et al; J Neurosci Res 2011; 89(9): 1499-508

19    Li, L et al;  Sci Rep 2014; 4: 6234

20    http://www.pubs.acs.org/doi/abs/10.1021/jf200379c

21    https://www.ncbi.nlm.nih.gov/pubmed/21910124

22    Bassirs-Jahromi S. Punica granatum (Pomegranate) activity in health promotion and cancer prevention. Oncol Rev. 2018; 12(1):345

23    Adaramoye O, Erguen B. Nitzsche B et al. Punicalagin, a polyphenol from pomegranate fruit, induces growth inhibition and apoptosis in human PC-3 and LNCaP cells. Chem Biol Interact. 2017; 274: 100-6.

24    Liu H, Zeng Z, Wang S et al. Main components of pomegranate, ellagic acid and luteolin, inhibit metastasis of ovarian cancer by down-regulating MMP2 and MMP9. Cancer Biol Ther. 2017; 18(12): 990-9.

25    Estrada-Luna D, Martinez-Hinojosa E, Cancino-Diaz JC, et al. Daily supplementation with fresh pomegranate juice increases paraoxonase 1 expression and activity in mice fed a high-fat diet. Eur J Nutr. 2018; 57(1):383-9.

26    https://www.ncbi.nlm.nih.gov/pmc/articles/PMC5806496/

27    https://www.ncbi.nlm.nih.gov/pubmed/22070054

28    https://www.eurekalert.org/pub_releases/2015-6/uow-amh061515.php

29    https://www.ncbi.nlm.nih.gov/pubmed/19373608

## Chapter 6

1    Bhori M, Singh K, et al. Exploring the effect of Vitamin E in Cancer Chemotherapy – A Biochemical and Biophysical Insight. J Biophotonics. 2018 May 16: e201800104.

2    www.drsimone.com

3    https://www.sciencedirect.com/science/articles/abs/pii/S075333 2298800887

4    https://www.canceractive.com/cancer-active-page-link.aspx?n=535&title=Beta-carotene

5    https://www.ncbi.nlm.nih.gov/pubmed/15557412?dopt=Abstract

6    Lappe et al. Journal of The American College of Nutrition. 2006;

25(5): 395-402

7    https://thetruthaboutcancer.com/vitamin-d-natures-medicine-chest

8    Holick, M.F. Mayo Clin Proc. 2006; 81:353-73.

9    Grant, WB and Hollick MF. Alt Med Review 2005 10(2): 94-111.

10   https://www.ncbi.nlm.nih.gov/pubmed/16380576

11   https://www.ncbi.nlm.nih.gov/pubmed/19470790

12   https://ar.iiarjournals.org/content/34/3/1163.full

13   Woo, TCS et al. Nutr Cancer. 2005; 51: 32-36

14   Moertel, CG et al, N Eng J. Med; vol 312 p. 137, 1985

15   Cameron, E, Pauling, L. Cancer Research. Vol 39 p. 663, March 1979.

16   Kock, CJ et al; J Cell Physial vol 94, p 299, 1978

17   https://www.cell.com/cancer-cell/fulltext/S1535-6108(17)30062-4

18   Maggini S1, Wintergerst ES, Beveridge S, Hornig DH. Selected vitamins and trace elements support immune function by strengthening epithelial barriers and cellular and humoral responses. Br J Nutr. 2007 Oct; 98 Suppl 1:S29-35.

19   Candeias SM1, Gaipl US. The Immune System in Cancer Prevention, Development and Therapy. Anticancer Agents Med Chem. 2016;16(1):101-7.

20   Prasad KN, Hernandez C, Edwards-Prasad J, Nelson J, Borus T, Robinson WA: Modification of the effect of tamoxifen, cisplatin, DTIC, and interferon-alpha 2b on human melanoma cells in culture by a mixture of vitamins. Nutr Cancer 22: 233-245, 1994.

21   Kurbacher CM, Wagner U, Kolster B, Andreotti PE, Krebs D, Bruckner HW: Ascorbic acid (vitamin C) improves the antineoplastic activity of doxorubicin, cisplatin, and paclitaxel in human breast carcinoma cells in vitro. Cancer Lett 103: 183-189, 1996.

22   https://www.pcrm.org/health/cancer-resources/diet-cancer/nutrition/how-vitamin-e-helps-protect-against-cancer.

23   The Blaylock Wellness Report, Vol 13, No. 9 (Sept 2016).

24   Springett GM et al. E Bio Medicine 2015; 2 (12):1987-95

25   Rahman AA et al; Molecules 2014; 19(9):14528-41

26   Miya-zawa T et al. Asia Pac J Clin Nutr 2008; 17: Suppl 1: 253-6

27   https://www.researchgate.net/publication/51807285_Tocotrienol_as_a_potential_anticancer_agent

28   https://www.ncbi.nlm.nih.gov/pubmed/19367124

29    Sokol RJ in PRESENT KNOWLEDGE IN NUTRITION p. 132 Ziegler ILSI Wash DC 1996

30    https://www.ncbi.nlm.nih.gov/pmc/articles/PMC5502190/

31    J Amer Med Assoc, Vol 244, p. 1077, 1980

32    https://www.ncbi.nlm.nih.gov/pmc/articles/PMC3250530/

33    https://www.ncbi.nlm.nih.gov/pubmed/18546288

34    https://www.onlinelibrary.wiley.com/doi/abs/10.1002/ijc.25546

35    https://www.nutraingredients-usa.com/Article/2016/07/19/Only-1-5-global-population-meet-ideal-vitamin-E-levels-Review

36    https://annals.org/aim/fullarticle/718049/meta-analysis-high-dose-vitamin-e-supplementation-may-increase-all

37    Krinsky, NI. Amer J Clin Nutr. Vol 53, p 238, 1991

38    Zhang, L et al; Carcinogenesis. Vol. 12, p. 2109, 1991

39    https://www.myactive8.com/HeatthUpdate_week0924Betacarotene_immune.htm

40    Bertram J.S et al; Nutrients and Cancer Prevention, Prasad KN (eds) p. 99 Humana 1990

41    https://ods.od.nih.gov/factsheets/VitaminA-HealthProfessional/

42    https://www.ncbi.nlm.nih.gov/pubmed/17284749

43    Zhang, XM et al; Virchows Archive. B Cell. Pathol. Vol 61, p 375, 1992

44    Fleet JC. Dietary selenium repletion may reduce cancer incidence in people at high risk who live in areas with low soil selenium. Nutr. Rev. 1979 Jul. 55(7): 277-9

45    https://www.ncbi.nlm.nih.gov/pubmed/21717786

46    https://www.ncbi.nlm.nih.gov/pubmed/18537721

47    Boik, J. "Zinc: Dietary Micronutrients and Their Effects on Cancer". Cancer and Natural Medicine (Princeton, MN: Oregon Medical Press, 1995), 147.

48    https://www.ncbi.nlm.nih.gov/pubmed/17344507

49    https://www.ncbi.nlm.nih.gov/pubmed/20155630

50    https://www.dailytargum.com/article/2014/10/researchers-discover-a-way-to-halt-cancer-now-thats-metal-c402

51    https://en.wikipedia.org/wiki/p53

52    https://www.fasebj.org/doi/abs/10.1096/fj.201700227rrr

53    https://beatcancer.org/blog-posts/magnesium

54    Bois, P. (1964) Tumour of the Thymus in Magnesium-deficient Rats. Nature. 204(1): p 1316

55    Seelig, MS in ADJUVANT NUTRITION IN CANCER TREATMENT, p. 284 Cancer Treatment Research Foundation (1994)

56    https://www.mgwater.com/Magnesium%20and%20Cancer.pdf

57    https://www.ncbi.nlm.nih.gov/pubmed/22854408

58    https://www.ncbi.nlm.nih.gov/pmc/articles/PMC3931212/

59    https://www.ncbi.nlm.nih.gov/pubmed/18796350

60    Johnstone TC et al. "Understanding and improving platinum anticancer drugs – phenathriplatin". Anticancer Research, 2014, 34(1): 471-476; PMID: 24403503, PMCID: PMC3937549

61    Hodgkinson, E et al; "Magnesium depletion in patients receiving cisplatin-based chemotherapy". Clinical Oncology (Royal College of Radiologists), 2006 Nov, 18(9): 710-8, PMID: 17100159

62    https://www.naturalmedicinejournal.com/journal/2014-06/iodine-and-cancer

63    Ghent, WR et al. Cancer J Surg. Vol 36, p. 453, 1993

64    https://thetruthaboutcancer.com/iodine-deficiency-cancer/

65    https://www.ncbi.nlm.nih.gov/pubmed/8127329

# Chapter 7

1    https://www.ncbi.nlm.nih.gov/pubmed/12611564

2    Chang, H. And But, P. Pharmacology and Applications of Chinese Materia Medica, Vol. 2, World Scientific, Singapore (1987)

3    Boik, J. CANCER AND NATURAL MEDICINE, p. 177, Oregon Medical, Princeton, MN, (1995)

4    Chan, T. Ancient Remedies Clues to Cancer. Health Freedom News 3:5 (1984)

5    Cha, R.J et al; Chung-Hua, Nei Ko Tsa Chit 33, p. 462 (1994)

6    Li, N.Q, Chung-Kuo, Chung Hsi I Chieh Ho Tsa Chih, Vol 12, p 588 (1992)

7    Cho, WC, Leung K.N. In vitro and in vivo anti-tumour effects of Astragalus membranaceus. Cancer Lett. July 8 2007; 252 (1): 43-54

8    Hsu HY, Oriental Materia Medica: A Concise Guide. Long Beach CA; Oriental Healing Arts Institute 1986

9    Higashitanai A, et al: Plant saponins can affect DNA recombination in cultured mammalian cells. Cell Struct Funct 1989; 14: p. 617-24

10    https://www.ncbi.nlm.nih.gov/pubmed/11532854

11    https://www.dynamicchiropractic.com/mpacms/dc/article.php?id=9456

12    https://www.ncbi.nlm.nih.gov/pubmed/12470437

13    https://www.mskcc.org/cancer-care/integrative-medicine/herbs/scuttellaria-baicalensis#field-herb-mechanism-of-action

14    Small EJ, Frohlich MW, Bok R, Shinohara K, Grossfeld G, Rozenblat Z, et al: Prospective trial of the herbal supplement PC-SPES in patients with progressive prostate cancer. J Clin Oncol 2000 Nov 1; vol 18(21): p 3595-603

15    Dzink JL, Socransky SS. Comparative in vitro activity of sanguinarine against oral microbial isolates. Antimicrob Agents Chemother 1985; 27(4): p 663-665

16    Mazzio EA, Soliman KF. In vitro screening for the tumouricidal properties of international medicinal herbs. Phytother Res 2009 March; 23(3): p 385-398

17    Han MH, Yoo YH, Choi YH. Sanguinarine-induced apoptosis in human leukemia U937 cells via BcL-2 downregulation and caspase-3 activation. Chemotherapy 2008; 54(3): p 157-165

18    Ding Z, Tang SC, Weerasinghe P, et al: The alkaloid sanguinarine is effective against multidrug resistance in human cervical cells via bimodal cell death. Biochem Pharmacol 2002; 63(8): p 1415-1421

19    https://www.ncbi.nlm.nih.gov/pubmed/26798435

20    https://www.ncbi.nlm.nih.gov/pubmed/10587640

21    https://www.ncbi.nlm.nih.gov/pubmed/22588059

22    Basini G, Santini SE, Bussolati S et al: Sanguinarine inhibits VEGF-induced Akt phosphorylation. Ann NY Acad Sci 2007; 1095; p 371-376

23    Eun JP, Koh GY. Suppression of angiogenesis by the plant alkaloid, sanguinarine Biochem Biophys Res Commun 2004; 317(2): p 618-624

24    Burgeiro A, Bento AC et al: Rapid human melanoma cell death induced by sanguinarine through oxidative stress. Eur J Pharmacol 2013 Apr 5; 705(1-3): 109-18

25    Lee JS, Jung WK, Jeong MH, Yoon TR, Kim HK. Sanguinarine induces apoptosis of HT-29 human colon cancer cells via the regulation of Bax/BcL-2 ratio and caspase-9-dependent pathway.

Int J of Toxicology. 2012; 31(1): 70-77

26    Van Wyk BE, Albrecht C. A review of the taxonomy, ethnobotany, chemistry and pharmacology of Sutherlandia fructescens (Fabaceae). J Ethnopharmacol Oct 28 2008; 119(3): 620-629

27    Tai J, Cheung S, Chan E, Hasman D. In vitro culture studies od Sutherlandia frutescens on human tumour cell lines, J Ethnopharmacol. July 2004; 93(1): 9-19

28    Chinkwo KA. Sutherlandia frutescens extracts can induce apoptosis in cultured carcinoma cells. J Ethnopharmacol. Apr 8 2005; 98(1-2): 163-170

29    Stander A, Marais S, Stivaktas V, et al. In vitro effects of Sutherlandia frutescens water extracts on cell numbers, morphology, cell cycle progression and cell death in a tumourigenic and a non-tumourigenic epithelial breast cell line. J Ethnopharmacol. July 6 2009; 124(1): 45-60

30    Grandi M RL, Vernay M Lessertia. (Suntherlandia frutescens) and fatigue during cancer treatment. Phytotherapie 2995; 3:110

31    https://www.sutherlandia.org/cancer

32    Sandoval M, Charbonnet RM, Okuhama NN, Roberts J, Krenova Z, Trentacosti AM, Miller MJ. Cat's claw inhibits TNF-alpha production and scavenges free radicals: role in cytoprotection. Free Radic Biol Med 2000; 29(1): 71-8

33    Garcia Prado E, Garcia Gimenez MD, De la Puerta Vazquez R et al. Anti-proliferative effects of mitraphylline a pentacyclic oxindole alkaloid of Unacaria tomentosa on human glioma and neuroblastoma cell lines. Phytomedicine Apr 2007; 14(4): 280-284

34    Pilarski R, Poczekaj-Kostrzewska M, Ciesiolka D et al. Antiproliferative activity of various Uncaria tomentosa preparations on HL-60 promyelocytic leukaemia cells. Pharmacol Rep. Sept-Oct 2007; 59(5): 565-572

35    Garcia Gimenez D, Garcia Prado E, Saenz Rodriguez T et al. Cytotoxic effect of the pentacyclic oxindole alkaloid mitraphylline isolated from Uncaria tomentosa bark on human Ewing's sarcoma and breast cancer cell lines. Planta Med. Feb 2010; 76(2): 133-136

36    Steinberg PN, "Cat's claw Update: Wondrous Herb from the Peruvian Rain Forest" Townsend Letter for Doctors and Patients (Aug/Sept 1995) 70-71

37    Dreifuss AA, Bastos-Pereira AL, Fabossi IA et al. Uncaria tomentosa

exerts extensive anti-neoplastic effects against the Walker-256 tumour by modulating oxidative stress and not by alkaloid activity. PLoS One. 2013; 8(2): e54618

38    https://www.ncbi.nlm.nih.gov/pubmed/11724307

39    Santos Araujo Mdo C, Farias IL, Gutierres J et al. Uncaria tomentosa-adjuvant treatment for breast cancer: clinical trial. Evid Based Complement Altermat Med. 2012; 2012: 676984

40    https://www.ncbi.nlm.nih.gov/pubmed/16445836

41    De Paula LC, et al. Uncaria tomentosa improves quality of life in patients with advanced solid tumours. J Altern Complement Med. 2015; 21(1): 22-30

42    Van Beek TA et al. Ginkgo biloba L. Fitoterapia 1998; 69: 195-244

43    https://www.mskcc.org/cancer-care/integrative-medicine/herbs/ginkgo

44    Bennett, SA et al. "Platelet Activating Factor, an Endogenous Mediator of Inflammation, Induces Phenotypic Transformation of Rat Embryo Cells" Carcinogenesis 14: 7 (1993), 1289-1296

45    Su AH Chen et al: Therapeutic mechanism of ginkgo biloba exocarp polysaccharides on gastric cancer. World J Gastroenterol 2003 Nov; 9(11): 2424-7

46    Kim ES, Rhee KH et al. Ginkgo biloba extract (EGb 761) induces apoptosis by the activation of caspase-3 in oral cavity cancer cells. Oral Oncol 2005 Apr; 41(4): 383-9

47    Ye B, Cramer D. Ginkgo biloba may helpprotect against ovarian cancer. Environmental Nutrition 01-Jan-06, Online

48    https://sciencedirect.com/science/article/pil/089158499400220E?via%3Dihub

49    Yang CS, etal: J Natl Cancer Inst. Vol 85 p 1038 (1993)

50    Cabrera C, Artacho R, Gimenez R. Beneficial effects of green tea – a review. Journal of the American College of Nutrition 2006; 25(2): 79-99

51    Ho C et al: Prev Med, vol 21 p 520, (1992)

52    https://www.ncbi.nlm.nih.gov/pubmed/15585768

53    https://www.ncbi.nlm.nih.gov/pubmed/10607735

54    https://www.ncbi.nlm.nih.gov/pubmed/14519824

55    https://www.ncbi.nlm.nih.gov/pubmed/?term=12121824

56    https://cancer.gov/about-cancer/causes-prevention/risk/diet/tea-fact-sheet

57 Kurahashi N, Sasazuki S, Iwasaki M, Inoue M, Shoichiro Tsugane for the JSG. Green Tea Consumption and Prostate Cancer Risk in Japanese Men: A Prospective Study. Am J Epidemiol 2007; 167(1): 71-77

58 https://www.ncbi.nlm.nih.gov/pubmed/16424063

59 Inoue M, Tajima K, Mizutani M et al: Regular consumption of green tea and the risk of breast cancer recurrence: follow-up study from the Hospital-based Epidemiologic Research Program at Aichi Cancer Center (HERPACC) Japan. Cancer Letters 2001; 167(2): 175-182

60 https://www.ncbi.nlm.nih.gov/pubmed/16311246

61 https://www.ncbi.nlm.nih.gov/pubmed/17548688

62 https://www.ncbi.nlm.nih.gov/pmc/articles/PMC2577676

63 https://www.ncbi.nlm.nih.gov/pubmed/?term=10918460

64 https://www.ncbi.nlm.nih.gov/pubmed/14518774

65 Rao K, et al: Cancer Res 28, 1952 (1968)

66 De Santana C, et al: Revista do Instituto de Antibioticos Recife 8, p 89 (1968)

67 Santana CF et al: Rev Inst Antibiot, (1980/81) 20, 61-68

68 Linardi, M.D.C et al "A Lapachol Derivative Active Against Mouse Lymphocyte Leukemia P-388". Journal of Medicinal Chemistry 18: 11 (1975), 1159-1162

69 https://www.ncbi.nlm.nih.gov/pubmed/15643520

70 Hu S.Y. "The Genus Panax (Ginseng) in Chinese Medicine". Economic Botany 30: 1 (1976), 11-18

71 Fulder S. The Root of Being, Hutchinson and Co, London 1980

72 Murray MT. Healing Power of Herbs, p 265, Prima Publ, Rocklin, CA 1995

73 https://www.cmjournal.org/content/pdf/1749=8546-2-6,pdf

74 Yamamoto M et al: Arzneim-Forsch 27, p 11 (1977)

75 Chen X: Abs Chin Med 3 p 91 (1989)

76 Shistar E, Sievenpiper JL et al: "The effect of ginseng (the genus panax) on glycemic control: a systematic review and meta-analysis of randomized controlled clinical trials" PLoS one, 2014 Sep 29; 9(9)

77 Zhou JC et al: Cancer Res Prev Treat 14, 149 (1987) in Abst Chin Med 2, 323 (1988)

78 Liu CX and Xiao PG: J Ethnopharmacol 36, 27 (1992)

79 Yun T and Choi S. "Preventative effect of ginseng intake against

various human cancers: a case-control study on 1987 pairs",
Cancer Epidemiology Biomarkers and Prevention, vol 4, no 4 p 401-
408, 1995

80   Cui Y, Shu XO, Gao YT et al: "Association of ginseng use with
     survival and quality of life among breast cancer patients". Am J
     Epidemial 163(7): p 645-653 (2006)

81   Liu CX and Xiao PG: J Ethnopharmacol 36, 27 (1992)

82   Brekhman II and Dardymov IV. Ann Rev Pharmacol 9 p 419, (1969)

83   Fulder S. The Root of Being, Hutchinson and Co, London 1980

84   Aggarwal, BB et al; Anticancer Res 2003; 23: 363-398

85   http://www.greenmedinfo.com/article/curcumin

86   http://www.greenmedinfo.com/article/efficacy-liposomal-curcumin

87   https://www.theatlantic.com/health/archive/2011/09/turmeric

88   http://www.greenmedinfo.com/article/curcumin

89   Khafif, A et al; Laryngoscope 2009; 119: 2019-2026

90   http://www.cancerresearchuk.org/about-cancer/cancers-in-
     general/cancer-questions/can-turmeric

91   Weng G et al. Biomed Res Int 2015; 2015.630397

92   Baharuddin, P et al. Oncol Rep 2016; 35: 13-25

93   Zhou Q et al. PLoS One 2015; 10: e0126694

94   Saha S et al. Anticancer Res 2012; 32: 2567-84

95   Thomas, Richard. The Essiac Report: Los Angeles. The Alternative
     Treatment Information Network. 1993

96   Olsen, Cynthia Essiac: A Native Herbal Cancer Remedy. Pagosa
     Springs, CO: Kali Press 1996

97   I was Canada's Cancer Nurse – The Story of ESSIAC by Rene M.
     Caisse.  www.essiacinfo.org/essiacstory.pdf

98   https://www.healthfreedom.info/cancer%20Essiac.htm

99   Walters, R. "Essiac". Options: The Alternative Cancer Therapy Book
     ( Garden City, NY: Avery Publishing, 1993) p 110

100  Moss, R. Cancer Therapy: The Independent Consumer's Guide (
     New York: Equinox Press, 1992

101  Moss, R. Herbs against Cancer: New York: Equinox Press 1998

102  https://www.alternative-cancer-care.com/essiac-tea-and-
     cancer.html

103  https://www.healthfreedom.info/cancer%20Essiac.htm

104  Glum, Gary. Calling of an Angel. Los Angeles: Silent Walker
     Publishing 1988

105 Goldberg, Burton. Alternative Medicine Definitive Guide to Cancer. California, Future Medicine Publishing 1997 p. 65

106 Boik, John. Natural Compounds in Cancer Therapy. Oregon Medical Press, 2001

107 Hoxsey, H.M. You Don't Have to Die (New York, NY: Milestone Books, 1956)

108 Ausubel, Kenny and Salveson, Catherine. Hoxsey: "How Healing Became a Crime". 87 minute documentary film. New York: Wellspring Media 1987

109 Fitzgerald, B.F. "A Report to the Senate Interstate Commerce Committee on the Need for Investigation of Cancer Research Organizations", Congressional Record, August 3, 1953, Vol. 99, Part 12, A5350-A5353, ( Washington, DC: US Government Printing Office, 1953)

110 https://www.canceractive.com/article/Hoxsey

111 Chowka, P.B. "Does Mildred Nelson Have an Herbal Cure for Cancer?" Whole Life Times pp. 16-18, Jan/Feb. 1984

112 Duke, J. "The Herbal Shotgun Shell" American Botanical Council's HerbalGram, No. 18/19, Fall 1988/Winter 1989, pp. 12-13

113 Spain-Ward, P. "History of Hoxsey Treatment", contract report submitted to U.S. Congress, Office of Technology Assessment, May 1988, p. 8

114 Bio-Medical Centre, Information sheet on Hoxsey Therapy, typescript, undated.

# Chapter 8

1 https://www.ncbi.nlm.nih.gov/pmc/articles/PMC4266698/

2 https://www.ncbi.nlm.nih.gov/pubmed/17024588/

3 https://www.ncbi.nlm.nih.gov/pmc/articles/PMC2664784/

4 https://www.sciencedirect.com/science/article/pii/S2221169115001446/

5 https://www.biomedcentral.com/content/pdf/1472-6882-12-253.pdf

6 https://www.ncbi.nlm.nih.gov/pubmed/26514509/

7 https://www.oapublishinglondon.com/articles/656

8     https://www.ncbi.nlm.nih.gov/pubmed/21287538

9     https://thetruthaboutcancer.com/essential-oils-for-cancer

10    https://thetruthaboutcancer.com/myrrh

11    https://www.ncbi.nlm.nih.gov/pubmed/26666387/

12    https://academicjournals.org/article1380545334Su%20et%20al.pdf

13    https://www.ncbi.nlm.nih.gov/pmc/articles/PMC3796379/

14    https://www.organicfacts.net/health-benefits/essential-oils/health-benefits-of-lavender-essential-oil.html

15    https://media.allured.com/documents/8459.pdf

16    https://thetruthaboutcancer.com/cancer-benefits-lavender-essential-oil/

17    https://www.ncbi.nlm.nih.gov/pubmed/26861249

18    https://www.ncbi.nlm.nih.gov/pubmed/25973472

19    https://www.ncbi.nlm.nih.gov/pubmed/24571090

20    https://www.ncbi.nlm.nih.gov/pmc/articles/PMC4142939/

21    https://www.ncbi.nlm.nih.gov/pmc/articles/PMC4497427

22    https://www.ncbi.nlm.nih.gov/pubmed/22895026

23    https://www.sciencedirect.com/science/article/pii/s094471131205120

24    https://www.nutrition-and-you.com/lemongrass.html

25    https://www.ncbi.nlm.nih.gov/pmc/articles/PMC3217679

26    https://www.ncbi.nlm.nih.gov/pubmed/15931590

27    https://www.ncbi.nlm.nih.gov/pubmed/15931590

28    https://www.researchgate.net/publication/265842609_Anticancer_effect_of_lemongrass_oil_and_citral_on_cervical_cancer_cell_lines

29    https://www.ncbi.nlm.nih.gov/pubmed/19121295

30    https://phcogfirst.com/sites/default/files/PC_3_4_6.pdf

31    https://www.ncbi.nlm.nih.gov/pubmed/?term=lemongrass+essential+oil+cancer

32    https://www.jpsr.pharmainfo.in/Documents/Volumes/vol6issue03/jpsr06031401A.p

33    https://www.ncbi.nlm.nih.gov/pmc/articles/PMC3449592

34    https://www.ncbi.nlm.nih.gov/pmc/articles/PMC3261448

35    https://www.ncbi.nlm.nih.gov/pubmed/20096548

36    https://www.ncbi.nlm.nih.gov/pubmed/19373612

37    https://www.mdpi.com/1420-3049/15/5/3200

38  https://www.ncbi.nlm.nih.gov/pubmed/24737278
39  https://www.aromatools.com/books-media/books-brochures/modern-essentials.html
40  https://www.tandfonline.com/doi/abs/10.1080/10412905.2003.9712248
41  https://www.ncbi.nlm.nih.gov/pubmed/21382660
42  https://www.ncbi.nlm.nih.gov/pmc/articles/PMC5133115
43  https://onlinelibrary.wiley.com/doi/abs/10.1111/j.1362-2672.1994.tb01661.x
44  https://www.ncbi.nlm.nih.gov/pubmed/20657472
45  https://www.tandfonline.com/doi/abs/10.1080/01635581.2012.719658?journalCode=hnuc20#.VRnVYWbqITn
46  https://www.ncbi.nlm.nih.gov/pubmed/9492350
47  https://www.ncbi.nlm.nih.gov/pubmed/26437948
48  https://www.researchgate.net/publication/269492503_Thyme

# Chapter 9

1  https://www.tcmworld.org/what-is-tcm/the-five-major-organ-systems/
2  https://www.bachcentre.com/centre/download/healers.pdf
3  https://www.mayoclinic.org/healthy-lifestyle/stress
4  Boik, John. Cancer and Natural Medicine: A Textbook of Basic Science and Clinical Research, Oregon Medical Press, 1996
5  https://www.godandscience.org/apologetics/smj.pdf
6  https://annals.org/aim/article-abstract/713514/efficacy-distant-healing-systematic-review-randomized-trials?volume=132&issue=11&page=903
7  Koenig HG. Religion, spirituality & health: the research & clinical implications. ISRN Psychiatry 2012 Dec 16; 2012: 278730
8  https://www.alternative-doctor.com/soul_stuff/prayermorrow.htm
9  https://www.catholicculture.org/culture/liturgicalyear/prayers/view.cfm?id=1307

# Chapter 10

1    https://budwigcenter.com
2    https://www.sciencedaily.com/releases/2017/11/171106121300.htm
3    https://blogs.scientificamerican.com/observations/cannabis
4    https://cbd-international.net/cannabis
5    https://www.spandidos-publications.com/10.3892/ijo.2017.4022
6    https://www.cancer.gov/about-cancer/treatment/cam/patient/cannabis
7    https://www.ncbi.nlm.nih.gov/pubmed/25916739
8    https://www.eurekalert.org/pub_releases/2018-04/eb2-hsp041318.php
9    https://www.cancer.gov/about-cancer/treatment/cam/patient/cannabis
10   https://www.ncbi.nlm.nih.gov/pubmed/25660577
11   https://www.ncbi.nlm.nih.gov/pubmed/30061636
12   http://mct.aacrjournals.org/content/early/2014/11/12/1535-7163.MCT-14-0402
13   https://www.ncbi.nlm.nih.gov/pmc/articles/PMC3202504/
14   https://www.ncbi.nlm.nih.gov/pubmed/21749363
15   Deitch, EA. Archives Surgery, vol 125, p 403, March 1990
16   https://www.ncbi.nlm.nih.gov/pubmed/15828052
17   https://medicalxpress.com/news/2016-02-probiotics-modulate-liver
18   https://www.medicalnewstoday.com/articles/319688.php
19   https://www.ncbi.nlm.nih.gov/pubmed/19423769
20   https://www.theguardian.com/society/2018/may/07/cancer-if-exercise-was-a-pill-it-would-be-prescribed-to-every-patient
21   Cherry, T. A theory of cancer. Med. J. Aust. 1: 425-438, 1922
22   Sivertsen, I., A.W. Dahlstrom. The relation of muscular activity to carcinoma: a preliminary report. J. Cancer Res. 6: 365-378, 1922
23   https://journals.lww.com/acsm-msse/Fulltext/2003/11000/Physical_Activity_and_Cancer_Prevention_Data_from.7.aspx
24   https://www.theguardian.com/society/2018/may/07/cancer-if-exercise-was-a-pill-it-would-be-prescribed-to-every-patient
25   https://www.bmj.com/content/321/7274/1424.extract

26   Tilden J.H. 1926 Toxemia Explained:  The true interpretation of the cause of disease Denver, Colorado.

27   https://www.naturalnews.com/027338_chelation_health_blood.html

28   https://www.onlinelibrary.wiley.com/doi/abs/10.1002/ptr.1838

29   https://www.ncbi.nlm.nih.gov/pubmed/17571966

30   https://chlorophyllwater.com/pages/what-is-chlorophyll

31   https://www.ncbi.nlm.nih.gov/pubmed/22038065

32   https://academic.oup.com/jn/article/135/8/1995/4663938

33   https://www.researchgate.net/publication/43335937_antimicrobial_activity_of_chlorophyll-based_solution_on_candida

34   https://link.springer.com/article/10.1007%2Fs10753-011-9399-0?LI=true

35   https://www.ncbi.nlm.nih.gov/pubmed/14690798

36   https://www.ncbi.nlm.nih.gov/pubmed/23134462

37   https://www.ncbi.nlm.nih.gov/pubmed/23633807

38   https://www.ncbi.nlm.nih.gov/pubmed/24269837

39   https://www.ncbi.nlm.nih.gov/pubmed/23743830

# Glossary of Terms

**Angiogenesis** – the development of new blood vessels that support the growth of tumours.

**Anti–Angiogenesis** – inhibition of the growth of new blood vessels.

**Anticancer** – the ability of a compound to destroy cancer cells.

**Antineoplastic** – is a broad term that refers to any agent that fights against cancer in any way.

**Antioxidant** – A molecule capable of inhibiting the oxidation of other molecules such as free radicals which can start chain reactions that damage cells and lead to chronic disease including cancer.

**Antitumour** – inhibiting or preventing the formation or growth of tumours.

**Apoptosis**– is a process by which a cell engages in programmed cell death or cellular suicide. It is an important method of cellular control and any disruption of this process leads to abnormal growth.

**Bioavailability** – amount of the active ingredients of vitamins or minerals that are absorbed by the body.

**Cachexia** – The loss of muscle mass and body weight.

**Cancer** – is a general term for a group of more than 100 diseases characterized by uncontrolled and abnormal growth of cells in different parts of the body.

**Cancer Stem Cells** – The 'seed' cells or 'parent' cells that produce cancerous daughter cells that make up the bulk of a tumour. They are notoriously difficult to kill with conventional chemotherapy or radiation. They can renew the cancer by diving and cause the formation of other cell types that form tumours.

**Carcinogen/Carcinogenic** – Any substance or agent that can cause cancer.

**Chemotherapy** – a form of cancer treatment in which drugs are used to kill cancer cells.

**Chromosome** – A strand of DNA that is encoded with genes, which are the units of heredity. In most cells, humans have 22 pairs of these chromosomes plus the two sex chromosomes (XX in females and XY in males) for a total of 46.

**Chronic** – a disease or condition that persists over a long period of time.

**Clinical Trials** – Research studies that are set up using human volunteers to compare new cancer treatments with the standard or usual treatments.

**Cytotoxic** – An agent or substance that is toxic to cells. It can refer to the action of drugs on healthy cells but in this book more usually refers to the action of drugs or natural compounds on cancer cells.

**DNA** – deoxyribonucleic acid, a complex molecular structure that contains each individual's genetic code, which instructs every cell in the body how to develop, live and reproduce.

**Free radicals** – are a group of atoms that have unpaired electrons, giving them an unstable negative charge. Free radicals are formed when oxygen interacts with certain molecules. The greatest danger of free radicals once they are formed is when they react with components of a cell such as the DNA or cell membrance causing damage and increasing cancer risk. For this reason, antioxidants are necessary to buffer the body from the deleterious effects of these free radicals.

**Gene** – A single unit of genetic information, stored on twisting strands of DNA in every cell of the body. Strands of DNA are tightly coiled together around proteins to form chromosomes; these are the basic units of heredity.

**Genetic** – Inherited; having to do with information that is passed from parents to their children through DNA.

**Immune System** – a complex network of cells, tissues and organs that protect the body against disease-causing agents, such as viruses, bacteria, fungi and harmful substances from the environment.

**Inflammation** – the immune system response to injury, infection or other stimuli. Ideally it is short-lived and self-limiting. Chronic inflammation is ongoing and is known to promote disease such as cancer.

**InVitro** – study done in a test tube or petri dish using isolated cells.

**InVivo** – study done in a living organism (animal or person)

**Ketogenic Diet** – a diet that focuses on foods very low in carbohydrates, uses moderate but regular high-fibre vegetables, is rich in natural fats and uses low to moderate protein. This results in the production of ketones (small chain fatty acids) which cancer cells are unable to use for energy production and are toxic to cancer cells.

**Lymphatic System** – The network of small vessels, nodes and glands, which filters body fluids back to the blood for elimination. Also, working in conjuction with the immune system to rid the body of debris and pathogens.

**Metastasis** – the spread of cancer cells from the primary site to other parts of the body.

**Mitochondria** – the organelle that produces energy (ATP) inside a cell.

**Oncogene** – a gene that when activated can send messages to cancer cells to promote their growth and spread.

**Oncology** – The study of cancer. A doctor who specialises in cancer is called an oncologist.

**Pathogens** – An infectious organism that causes disease to its host.

**Phytochemical** – A chemical compound that occurs naturally in plants and is a term generally used to refer to those chemicals that may positively affect health.

**Phytonutrient** – the term used to describe plant compounds which have health-promoting qualities.

**Prebiotics** – substances that feed the good bacteria in the gut.

**Probiotics**–live microorganisms (bacteria) that are beneficial to the health and balance of the human gut. They are also called 'friendly' or 'good' bacteria.

**Prognosis** – the likely outcome or chances of surviving a disease.

**Radiation Therapy (Radiotherapy)** – Treatment with high-energy from x-rays or other sources to kill cancer cells.

**Tissue** – A collection of cells that work together to perform a certain job or function in the body. Different parts of the body, such as the skin, lungs, liver or nerves are comprised of tissue.

**Tumour** – An abnormal mass of tissue. A tumour can be cancerous, or it can be benign, meaning it is not cancerous.

**Tumour Suppressor Genes** – Genes in the body that can stop or block the development of cancer.

# INDEX

# D

# E

# F